RADIANT
AGAIN & FOREVER

RADIANT
AGAIN & FOREVER

With Bioidentical Hormones
and Other Secrets

Prudence Hall, MD

Foreword by Suzanne Somers

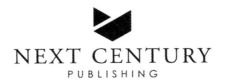

NEXT CENTURY
PUBLISHING

RADIANT
AGAIN & FOREVER
With Bioidentical Hormones and Other Secrets

Copyright ©2017 by Prudence Hall, MD
All rights reserved.

Published by Next Century Publishing
Austin, TX
www.NextCenturyPublishing.com

ISBN: 978-1-68102-171-3
Library of Congress: 2017932409

Printed in the United States of America

I dedicate this book to my children

Heston, Beryl and Conrad Liebowitz

&

To all women who seek the radiance of their own heart.

Gratitudes

Doron Libshtein, you stood by me as my mentor and friend for every word of this book. It was your penetrating understanding of what I wanted to convey and your inspiring presence that kept me on track. With your guidance and discernment, this book flowed from me, joyfully. You helped me plan all the chapters, create bullet points for the paragraphs, and listened to every word in our weekly mentoring sessions. After reading each section to you, your comments were so perceptive and interesting that I was inspired to rewrite everything with more depth. As the founder of "Mentors Channel" and the chairman of numerous companies, including The Hall Center, I know how busy you are. I give you my gratitude for magically suspending time for this book to come through. My heart literally overflows with love for the unique experience we shared during this process. Your masterful approach in helping me become a new writer and speaker will forever remain in my heart.

DL, my deepest gratitude.

Suzanne Somers, my fellow conspirator and darling friend, you are the one who gave me the "*secret formula*" to create a "*best-selling book.*" Having written best-selling sensations for decades, you have a clear understanding of this process and graced me with your knowledge. When I finally finished the first draft of my book and called to tell you the good news, you said, "Prudence, it sounds like a great book, but it's not the one we talked about you writing." LOL! You were right, it wasn't! So you talked to me again about how to approach my subject, and after another six months this book popped out, proving you to be absolutely right. My heart overflows with happiness for your splendid foreword and gratitude for your authenticity, kindness, courage, and all the ways you inspire me and millions of people to be their healthiest best. Over the years I have said how you deserve an honorary medical degree for all your groundbreaking work, and if those crazy medical schools don't jump on this, I am going to bequeath it to you from the hallowed halls of The Hall Center. Dr. Somers, I love you dearly!

Dearest Robin McGraw, you are always on the big stage, but even with your tireless work and inspiring foundations, you not only took the time to meet with me multiple times, but your contributions inspired me to add an additional chapter to this book—your glorious last chapter 12! Your self-knowledge and courage to be your authentic self touched and impressed me greatly. I cried when I re-read some of your stories. I speak with so many accomplished people, but your brilliance about life and your numerous revelations left me recommitted to my own values and self. We suffer, breakthrough to love, and then help others. That is how it works. Thank you my wonderful friend for helping make the world a better place, including your *When Georgia Smiled: Robin McGraw Revelation Foundation* for domestic violence. All of your good work and your significant contribution to this book touch me profoundly. My generous and radiant friend, I give you my heartfelt gratitude.

Karina Stewart, my dearest friend, not only is your life inspiring to me, but you have served as one of my formidable guides for many years. My warmest gratitude for your generous contribution to my book, and for co-founding *Kamalaya* with your husband John. You have both created heaven on earth with your wellness resort and what I consider to be my second home. With each visit I experience a healthier, more expanded sense of myself. Where am I writing this from now? *Kamalaya*! After pounding out the last part of this book, I needed Kamalaya's serenity and peace.

Radhanath Swami, dear one, just when I thought I had finished this book, Jeffrey Van Dyk gave me your book, *The Journey Home*. Big mistake! It immediately became one of my favorite books and the gold standard for this book. I was so touched and inspired by the way you generously shared your life's journey, that I spent many months rewriting countless passages in mine. Your magnificent new book, *The Inner Journey*, your generosity to mankind, and all of the ways you are in service, make this small gratitude to you one that comes straight from my heart. Thank you for inspiring me by following your own path of pure love and devotion.

Bette Light, dear wonder woman, I offer my gratitude for helping this book reach a greater audience and for your ideas and encouragement. You are a flow of creative understanding and have been so helpful over the past two years with all my projects. Your integrity is phenomenal, and I will tell anyone who is interested in being the best that, "You and your Light Years Ahead team are phenomenal!"

Richard Baskin, dear friend, thank you for your wise counsel over the years and for your brilliance in helping name *Radiant Again & Forever* the book. Love you.

Wendy Zahler, thank you for your magnificent help in the 10th hour when I really needed it. You have been so dear!

Simon Presland, thank you for your patient and steady editing and your skill in helping a new writer come out with her first book. It wasn't easy with my schedule and deadlines being missed, and I give you my true gratitude for standing by with encouragement and the "oomph" needed to bring this home. I also extend my warmest thanks to your wonderful Next Century Publishing team.

Kathryn and James B. Hall, my dearest sister and beloved father, you are the writers in this family, and it is such an honor to put this small offering next to your larger ones. Being born into a family of writers raises the bar and deepens the privilege of writing. Kathryn, over the years you have helped me with my poetry and this book with love, and you have been a shining example of what sisters can be for each other. My heart is wide open to you, and to our warrior father who wrote before us.

Elinor Venske, **Millicent Powers and James Hall**, I love and honor each of you, dear sibs, and feel a greater joy in life because of you. Elizabeth Hall, divine mother, you are part of each of us; my gratitude for your wisdom and for life.

Love and light,

Prudence

Table of Contents

RADIANT
AGAIN & FOREVER

Foreword

Hold onto your hats! If you are looking to regain quality of life and optimal health, you are going to find it here.

With my many books on health and natural bioidentical hormone replacement, this is the one book I couldn't write. I'm not able to take my readers into the examining room but that is exactly where Dr. Prudence Hall takes you. I can get you to the right door, I can empower you with information, I can teach you how your body works (or isn't working) but after that it has to be about being with the right doctor.

In the fast moving, cutting-edge world of bioidentical hormone replacement, going to a doctor who hasn't versed him or herself in real, natural bioidentical hormone replacement is like going to a plumber for a heart bypass. It's that out of their realm.

Dr. Hall is the right doctor, well versed and an expert, and now she is graciously going to allow you to be a "fly on the wall" in her examination room, listening in and observing. You will realize You Are Not Alone, that your problems are common to many women experiencing this "change," that your confusion and frustration is understandable and, best of all, it's fixable.

Dr. Hall will fix your husband also.

I try to infuse my readers with knowledge and confidence, so when meeting with a qualified doctor such as Dr. Hall they can get to work immediately and not have to start at "kindergarten." The more knowledge you have about how your body works (or doesn't), the sooner you will be able to start the reversal process. Knowledge is power and anyone enduring the suffering of hormonal decline needs to understand that quality of life is theirs, if this is done correctly. Women and men alike want to put their lives back together again and regain optimal health and quality of life, and that is what Dr. Hall's protocol offers.

Prudence is my friend, my colleague and my doctor. I am grateful to know such a gifted, talented, qualified and fine person. She is the real deal. She understands the entire package, and as a searcher for truth she brings to her examining room a completely different experience than you will find in most doctors' offices.

In menopause herself, Dr. Hall discusses the confusions she has experienced before finding the bliss of balance. Imagine the advantage of working with someone who truly "gets it." This is an entire program, starting with deep compassion for your journey. She is not going to dismiss you or your symptoms. She understands that in today's world returning to balance is three pronged:

- First, replace hormones gradually to optimal levels as determined by lab work plus observances made during your initial consult. For instance, if you are missing the outer third of your eyebrows she will know intuitively that your thyroid is not in balance. This kind of detective work is extremely important because all hormones must be in balance. If one is off, then they are all off, and a qualified doctor knows this. There is no one-pill-fits-all.

- Second, explain that your toxic burden will affect your hormonal output or decline. Detoxification and building up important missing minerals and nutrients are crucial to finding perfect balance. Toxicity is blunting hormones at a rate never seen before in humanity.

- Third is the spiritual component: your thought-life creates, and negativity results in negativity. She will open you to the world of meditation and gratitude, to see that one door closing is not an end but a beginning. Finding true balance requires an understanding of the body/mind connection.

Hormone replacement opens a new way to experience the second half of life and make it enjoyable. Imagine enjoying aging! As you reach menopause you possess what no young person can have or buy: wisdom and perspective. In the fog of hormonal decline it's hard to access these two amazing gifts, but when the fog lifts, a new and brighter world is revealed, and this is what you can expect.

It's important to understand you are a critical part of the program. You must put in the work required. It took a long time to lose these hormones; it will take a while to build them back up—and it must be done gradually. Patience is required but if you hang in there, do what Dr. Hall says, take your diet seriously, work at sleeping eight hours nightly and find love and meaning, you will experience a fantastic ride.

I have experienced this bliss for the last twenty years, along with millions of other women and men. There is no underestimating quality of life. What good is having longevity without quality? It is extremely gratifying to see how many people have jumped onboard this fast-moving train and are now enjoying and luxuriating in this incredible journey. Once on this train you will never, ever look back.

Please note: Dr. Hall's advice is not conventional. For instance, perhaps lost libido can be jumpstarted again with hormone replacement and "twisting the nipples for five minutes" to release oxytocin, the love hormone. This will stimulate sensation, and increased oxytocin output relaxes, de-stresses—and no small thing, it feels good!

I realize this kind of "prescription" is a head-snapper and not the usual rap you get from a doctor, but this suggestion is a win/win for each partner. (What a nice assignment for a frustrated husband!) This is exactly what everyone loves about this woman—the unexpected. Sometimes we need a little shove and Dr. Hall knows when it is called for.

Dr. Hall is highly educated. She is a gynecologist and surgeon, hormone specialist, and a believer that to be healthy the human condition must be addressed as a major factor in achieving peak health. She has been exposed to the best and brightest minds. She is open, loving, and enthusiastic—and you, the patient, are the beneficiary. Nothing is off the table with her, so the patient feels comfortable and protected to tell her ANYTHING. In addition to her warmth and caring, you will feel that you've just made a new best friend.

Hormone replacement is more than restoration to perfect balance. The results will manifest as a return to the "you" that you used to be. Your beauty will return, your vitality will be restored and the internal "you" will achieve a state of health you may never have dreamed possible.

Prudence and I have known each other for many years, and I am proud of this book that she has written. It is a gift to you and to all of us.

Get ready…your life is about to change!

Suzanne Somers

Introduction

In writing this book, I want to offer women who are struggling with their health a new way of experiencing life—a transition *away from* the pain, suffering, confusion and health problems they are facing and *toward* a new happiness, youthful vitality, confidence, and natural radiance.

As a gynecologist for 30 years, I have helped more than 30,000 patients through the transitions and struggles so many women are currently facing. Over the years, I have developed unique and effective ways of approaching the hardest issues women deal with, bringing clarity and understanding to each problem.

As you read this book, you will realize that you are not alone on your journey to wholeness. In these pages you will find many others who suffer from similar symptoms and life circumstances as you do. Each chapter chronicles the journey I have taken with one of my patients going through a specific crisis such as menopause, the inability to lose weight, depression, anxiety, sexual problems, and sleeplessness. As the stories unfold with the challenges and symptoms of each client and the unique solutions I offer, I want you to glean possibilities for yourself. My approach encompasses a new style of medicine called *Regenerative Medicine,* which identifies the root causes of each client's symptoms and applies creative solutions based on hormonal balance, genetic composition, inflammatory triggers, toxic exposures and unique emotional problems.

As each woman tells her story, I want you to evaluate how your symptoms might be similar to hers. In fact, I want you to literally diagnose yourselves as well as your friends, sisters and mothers based on what you read. I will help you understand what is happening to your body and take charge of your life again. As women we are all in this together, and once you become healthy and whole again, I would love for you to become a guide and beacon for others.

Most doctors are not aware of the information I present in this book, so you might have to help your doctor arrive at your correct diagnosis. This is fair—please don't consider it to be pushy or arrogant. So many women have seen multiple doctors before finally getting the help they need! And it is shocking how many years these women suffered needlessly. I don't want you to go undiagnosed or untreated for a moment longer. In the same way an architect needs input before planning someone's dream house, good doctors very much need and appreciate the insight you can give them into your health. It's not difficult to become proficient regarding your own body, and it will be my honor to help you do just that!

This book will not only help with the health transitions you are facing, but also inspire you to see new possibilities for your life. I believe that true health is supported by three pillars: your physical body, the power of your mind with its thoughts and emotions, and your connection to your authentic self and your true life's purpose. When each of these is addressed, we become full of life, leaving any deadness behind. The results are explosive, igniting new vitality and union with your true self. You deserve to be fabulous! You deserve to love and be loved—to be happy and live a passionate life. Chapter after chapter will illustrate how eager my patients are to regain their health and energy. You will see how easily your physical reality can change, and how quickly a new life will spring forth.

I want you to receive everything you want in life, so let's begin …

Chapter 1

The Journey Out of Menopause

I am in the middle of a busy day when Julia walks into my consult room. I always look forward to meeting new clients. I give her a big welcome hug before she sits down on my Balinese sofa. I start our conversation by asking what is troubling her. Julia tries to speak—but her emotions are so overwhelming she puts her head in her hands and begins to sob.

I quietly reach out to touch her arm in sympathy. "I understand, honey. Sometimes it's all just too much. It can feel terrible, like you don't know who you are anymore. I would love to hear all about it."

Julia's need to tell her story is evident as the words begin to tumble chaotically from her mouth. "Seven years ago, I was happily married and successful in my job as a book editor. I loved helping my authors. Then, after the birth of my second child when I was thirty-nine, I started feeling ill. At first I thought I was just tired from the baby and work, but my condition steadily worsened. I felt depressed, exhausted, and all my muscles ached. I became so anxious I couldn't sleep.

"A few years ago it got so bad I had to stay in bed most of the day. My doctor told me I had fibromyalgia and prescribed Zoloft and pain meds. I was able to return to work again, and even though that was eight years ago, I still have to keep calling in sick all the time because I am just so exhausted. I know I'm going to lose my job … and maybe that's okay because I just can't do this anymore.

"I can't sleep! I wake up at three in the morning and just lie there. I've tried everything: Nyquil, Benadryl, all kinds of herbal things and even Ambien. Even if I'm able to sleep a few more hours, I still wake up feeling like I never went to bed. I drink a lot of coffee during the day to help me stay awake but it makes me feel jumpy.

"I'm so angry all the time. My poor kids and husband! I went from being such a good mom to being some kind of alien. My husband was patient at first, but this has been going on for seven years now, and I am only getting worse. It doesn't help that I've gained almost thirty pounds, so I'm fat on top of everything else. I don't even want to make love. Ever! I'm embarrassed to tell you this, but I've only made love a few times in the last year."

Julia cries again in earnest. "I am so ugly. How could this happen? I'm losing my husband. I have lost myself. I can't even think clearly anymore, and I'm so depressed I keep thinking about dying. Dr. Hall, I can't die and leave my children! I went to the emergency room twice this year with my heart pounding so hard I thought I was having a heart attack. Can you believe they told me I was having panic attacks? My doctor sent me to a psychiatrist who wanted to put me on a second antidepressant. I gained twelve pounds with the first one and I sure didn't want to gain more with a second one. I think I'm more depressed about gaining twelve pounds than I was before the Zoloft. I'm on sleeping meds, Xanax for panic attacks, and Zoloft for depression. I'm only forty-seven and it feels like my life is done. I just can't do this. Please help me. Please!"

I touch Julia's arm and search her eyes. She looks exhausted, her skin is dry, and her eyes and face look bloated. Her sagging arms catch my attention—the lack of muscle definition indicates her hormones are depleted. Julia's story could indicate a number of hormone abnormalities, but I hear such similar stories every day that it is actually very straightforward. Every symptom is typical of menopause, including the downward spiral she is describing. The only typical symptoms she didn't mention are hot flashes and night sweats, but approximately 40 percent of patients never experience those symptoms. Just to be sure, I ask her about it.

> *It is not at all uncommon for the menopause diagnosis to be missed because a woman still has periods and doesn't have the stereotypical presentation of hot flashes.*

"Nope," she replies. "I had a few four or five years ago, but nothing for years. I thought I was in menopause back then but my doctor disagreed. He said my symptoms started too early for that, and I still have my periods, so I guess I was wrong."

I sigh sympathetically. It is not at all uncommon for the menopause diagnosis to be missed because a woman still has periods and doesn't have the stereotypical presentation of hot flashes. In fact, menstrual periods frequently continue several years after menopause begins.

It takes some time for the clock to unwind. A five-second glance at Julia's lab values confirms she is definitely well into menopause and also has a pre-diabetic sugar level.

As I touch her arm I feel a kind of electric energy pulsing through her, which is typical of women in menopause—they are very anxious! They feel like they are missing a plane flight 24/7. The anxiety and suffering that Julia and so many other women go through is frustrating. Doctors should check a woman's hormone levels, no matter how old she is. Compassion rises within me. "Julia, you were right when you told your doctor years ago that you were in menopause. Let's review the evidence."

I give all new patients a binder containing their information. We open Julia's binder to discuss and explain her lab values, starting with her reproductive hormones. Her estrogen level is not just low, it is nonexistent. And her FSH is very high. An elevated FSH value (follicle-stimulating hormone) indicates that her brain is asking for more estrogen, because a woman's brain simply doesn't function well without it. When the FSH is higher than twenty, the diagnosis of menopause is clear. I draw Julia's values onto a menopause graph and watch the shock in her eyes when she sees how low her hormones are compared to normal.

"See? No doubt about it. Your levels indicate classic menopause."

Julia's body collapses a bit and then straightens up. "I knew I was in menopause, but no one listened; but I can't say I'm happy with *that* diagnosis either. In fact, I hate it! It feels old—as old as my grandmother. Can we fix it? Please, can we fix it?"

Julia begins to look hopeful when I explain that, while it will take a few months, we can bring her body out of that unhealthy menopausal state, which causes wicked symptoms and wreaks all kinds of havoc with the body's chemistry. When estrogen is low, inflammation, blood sugar, stress and cholesterol become elevated—and these are the root causes of most of the diseases of aging. It's like a teeter-totter. As soon as we raise a woman's estrogen, negative symptoms of aging and disease begin to decline.

> *When estrogen is low, inflammation, blood sugar, stress and cholesterol become elevated—and these are the root causes of most of the diseases of aging.*

"Oh, my God!" Julia exclaims, eyes wide with disbelief. "My doctor recently told me my cholesterol is high, and I have *never* had that before. And I feel so inflamed I know I am getting arthritis like my mom did. I had no idea menopause could cause all these symptoms. Now that you're telling me this, I remember reading Suzanne Somers' book, *I'm Too Young for This.* It was wonderful, but that was years ago and my brain just doesn't retain things like it used to." Julia's voice rises in distress. "Dr. Hall, I know this sounds like I'm making a joke about Suzanne's book, but I just get kind of a sick feeling about being in menopause; really, I think *I am* too young for this! Everyone knows menopause happens when you're old!"

Suzanne Somers has written multiple books about menopause, perimenopause, and cutting edge health solutions. She is a strong and perceptive spokesperson for my kind of medicine! Every week women come to me because of her books, crying with relief after they are helped and praising Suzanne as their personal angel. My prayers are that this book will also reach those in need and be another pillar of support for women.

The golden afternoon light floods the room as we continue our discussion. "Menopause can happen at any age, but the most common age is forty-four to forty-nine. In our mothers' generation it typically happened about five years later, but with all the stress and toxicity we are exposed to it now happens much earlier. I take care of so many women who are menopausal in their early forties. You're actually doing really well. You probably began perimenopause right after the birth of your baby at age thirty-nine. Most likely, menopause began in earnest three to four years ago when you started feeling really terrible. This diagnosis can be a shock for women. Were you hoping to have another baby?"

"I always wanted three children but since I've been so tired I feel lucky to have two, so that's not the problem. The problem is I'm aging so quickly. I feel I have become my mother. Men used to want my attention but now I have become almost invisible. And I hate myself because I can't stop eating. It's all my fault that I look like this."

I assure Julia that any "fault" was with her hormones.

> *Estrogen replacement prevents up to 50 percent of death from heart attacks.*

I explain that when we loose our hormones, we're like a plant in a dark closet without water or sunlight. Such a plant doesn't do so well, just like women don't do well without their proper hormone levels. Menopause is responsible for so many of the diseases that strike women as they age. Estrogen is anti-inflammatory, so when levels fall during menopause, arthritis and pain occur. Low estrogen is responsible for many women developing heart disease. In fact, heart attacks are the most common cause of death in women. When we replace our hormones with natural estrogen identical to our own estrogen, half of women's death from heart attacks are prevented. These natural estrogens are called bioidenticals, and they help us dial back the clock of aging. Healthy, youthful hormones result in healthy physiology. Not only are heart attacks prevented, but also dementia, diabetes and many cancers. It is also the best strategy to prevent osteoporosis and aging skin. I liken menopause to a woman's own personal tornado. It causes destruction as it passes through the body, wiping out good health, emotional stability, and frequently her relationships. It can also result in death.

"I do feel like I have a tornado inside, but won't this all stop after I go through menopause?"

I let out a deep breath. "Julia, it would be so nice if we could weather the storm of menopause naturally and end up on the other side in post-menopausal paradise, but that's not how it works. Unfortunately, once a woman is in menopause she stays there until she dies. Menopause is like spraying a fire hose on a house for years. The force of the water will eventually erode the structure and the house will fall. We need to rebalance your hormones and immediately get you out of menopause or else you will stay like you are now for the rest of your life. We need to prevent further problems and also repair the damage that's already been done."

A tiny, brave smile creases Julia's lips. "I feel like my structure has already totally collapsed and there's no one inside anymore. I disappeared with the house."

"We'll rebuild the house, I promise. Here's some good news. Your thyroid gland is still functioning quite well, and so are your adrenal hormones. Although they are a bit high, they haven't burned out yet. That's really good news, because so many women in menopause have deficiencies in every hormonal system. This means you still have some resilience left. The bioidentical hormones will help rebuild your body."

> *Hormones are your body's software.*

"I like the idea of using natural hormones," Julia responds, "but I heard hormones are dangerous and increase the risk of breast cancer. My grandmother died of that, so I might be at higher risk."

"Where did you hear that hormones are dangerous?" I ask.

"Well, everyone says they are, but it actually might be worth dying a few years earlier if I can feel better now. I mean, I don't want to go on living like this."

"That would be a *terrible* trade off," I respond. "I wouldn't accept that for myself or for any of my patients. There is no way I would be so pro bioidenticals if they *caused* more diseases, Julia. Proper hormone levels absolutely help women remain healthy and youthful."

I tell all of my patients the following about hormones:

- Hormones are your body's software. That's why I call my supplement line *Body Software*. When you turn on your computer it won't work unless its battery is charged and its software is loaded. The same is true of the body. Hormones are needed for every function it performs. Hormones make the heart beat, maintain blood pressure, and allow us to think, sleep, walk and breathe. Hormones repair cellular damage and prevent cancerous cells from growing. If we lost all our hormones we wouldn't live longer than about four minutes. As we age and hormone levels decline we get sick and the body doesn't function properly. When hormones and enzymes decline below a critical level, we die.

- It is of vital importance to keep hormone levels balanced at youthful levels. Old people have old hormones, and that's one of the reasons they get sick and lose their beautiful vitality.

- Premarin and other non-bioidentical hormones are *not* the same as bioidentical hormones. Premarin was manufactured before we had any idea that hormones even existed. Scientists tested all kinds of animal products and came up with the idea that using the urine of pregnant mares might help women in menopause. Well, it was a brave idea, but given that we didn't even have the word "hormone" in our medical vocabulary it was definitely a primitive beginning. It simply doesn't make sense that so many doctors still prescribe Premarin and Provera for the treatment of menopausal symptoms. We wouldn't consider a computer that's ten years old to be the best buy, yet doctors continue to use medical technology that is more than seventy-five years old in prescribing hormones for women.

> *Premarin and other non-bioidentical hormones are not the same as bioidentical hormones.*

- When I was just beginning my medical practice, the only hormones available were the non-bioidentical ones. My experience with prescribing synthetic hormones like Premarin and Provera was not good! Patients gained weight, felt bloated, and didn't feel much better than they did before I prescribed them.

- In 2001 a big study came out about Premarin and Provera that made me very happy. (I'd stopped prescribing them fifteen years earlier.) The Women's Health Initiative showed a marked increase in the incidences of breast cancer, heart attacks, dementia, blood clots and strokes among women who took synthetic hormones. Nevertheless, doctors still continue to prescribe them regularly.

- Bioidentical hormones come from soy and yams. They are created in high-tech labs to be identical to the hormones our body makes. You can analyze them with the most sophisticated tools available to medical science and you will find that they are exactly the same as the hormones made by the human body.

- Whether your body makes them or you take them it's the same thing—as long as you use bioidenticals.

- Back in the early 1980s, I started hearing about bioidentical hormones in Europe. I began prescribing them for my patients and they experienced huge improvements in terms of vitality, brain function, weight loss, beauty, sleep, and sex drive.

- As data emerged from large studies on bioidenticals, they showed as much as a 50 percent decrease in death from heart

> *Bioidentical hormones come from soy and yams. They are created in high-tech labs to be identical to the hormones our body makes.*

attacks and from dementia. Results also indicated fewer cases of diabetes, lowered cholesterol levels, lowered blood pressure, stronger bones, weight loss and much less depression. In short, the data on bioidenticals showed benefits for women on many levels.

- My personal experience with prescribing bioidenticals for more than 30 years is excellent. In my practice, where I prescribe bioidentical hormones for most of my patients, only three women have experienced a heart attack—and those were not fatal. Among my patients who take bioidentical hormones, breast cancer occurrences are 60 percent lower than average. These women remain strong, fit, sensual and beautiful as they age and do much better than patients who do not take bioidentical hormones.

- My motto for bioidentical hormones is this: Feel better, live longer.

As I continue my conversation with Julia, I assure her, "I have only a few patients out of thousands who don't feel better on estrogen cream. If you're one of them, we'll try a different approach. It takes a few weeks before you experience results, because the hormones need to get into your body and change your body chemistry and cells but most women do see a change. I'll have my patient educator explain exactly how to use the cream morning and evening. Now, let's talk sex." I laugh as I watch her perk up.

"Good! It's like I have a demon in my body destroying my relationship with my husband and men in general. Even if Brad Pitt were in the room today, I'd be totally turned off. Not that he would be interested in me," she moans. "I don't even want to think about sex. I was walking up some stairs the other day and my husband was following me. He reached out and put his hand on my butt, and I wanted to turn around and deck him. I felt such rage that I don't know how I controlled myself. It was awful!"

"I understand, Julia, and I want you to know you're not alone with this situation. Most of my patients in menopause and perimenopause tell me they are fed up with their partners and don't make love

> *Without testosterone, women lose muscle mass and the metabolic rate drops.*

often. In fact, that 'butt test' is a sure diagnosis of menopause. Unfortunately, not having a sex drive can harm many marriages. Women understand this and tell me all the time they feel sorry for their husbands, or that they fake it or have 'pity' sex. Menopause feels a bit like when we were prepubescent and thought boys were icky. That's how girls feel before their hormones kick in, and we go back to that state when we lose our hormones at menopause."

Julia's testosterone level is a paltry ten (when it should be at least fifty), which is a significant contributor to her low libido. Such a low level also decreases or eliminates a woman's ability to experience orgasm, which increases the feeling of inadequacy so many menopausal women experience. Recent studies show testosterone actually helps decrease breast cancer. That's a nice bonus for women.

I instruct Julia to use one click of the testosterone cream to the side of her body and a tiny dab of it right across the clitoris and the area between the vagina and rectum. Because muscle tone is weakened by menopause, Kegel exercises help get the orgasm muscles in shape.

"Julia, low testosterone also causes weight gain. Without testosterone, women lose muscle mass and the metabolic rate drops. Consider how quickly men lose weight. They pump a bit of iron and lose ten pounds in a few weeks. Why? Their testosterone levels are around 800, so they immediately rebuild their muscle, which raises their metabolism."

"I know!" Julia chimes in, "My husband looks great at forty-eight and doesn't struggle at all with his weight. I hate him! I'm starting to look like my mother. I am done with that! Prudence, I am getting myself back!"

Julia's marital situation has deteriorated to the point that she is considering a divorce. She is hurt and angry with her husband because he has distanced himself from her and is critical of the stranger she has become since menopause hit. I suggest we get her hormones in balance before she takes action to end her marriage. I promise her we won't ignore this elephant in the room. With so many of my clients, I have seen that menopause is a time for a woman to concentrate on herself—maybe for the first time in years. It might be that Julia and her husband won't stay together, or maybe they will fall back into each other's arms again. It can go either way during this huge life transition. Menopause forces a woman to stop and evaluate her life. Our needs become greater, and we have to take care of ourselves first. In a way, it's like putting on our own oxygen mask before helping others.

> *Menopause forces a woman to stop and evaluate her life. Our needs become greater, and we have to take care of ourselves first.*

"Your life is precious, and this time at the Center is for you. It's important to examine your life, to get in touch with who you really are and why you are here. Each stage of life reveals new insights and growth. You could live for another fifty years, and the longer you live, the more you can explore and develop. Do you see this playing out in your life?"

"Yes, my purpose has been raising my kids, volunteering, helping the school, and helping my husband. But I see it is all shifting. Maybe that's some of the anxiety I feel. I'm so anxious I can hardly even drive."

"Do you have any intuition about where this shift is taking you?"

"I have no idea. But I sometimes wake up in the middle of the night scared that I am going to die before I have ever really lived. Dr. Hall, I'm in a crisis, and it doesn't feel like it's only menopause."

"Julia, menopause is a physical change that causes emotional and life changes as well. You *are* in a kind of crisis, but it's one that offers a unique opportunity for greater expansion and expression. The leaves fall in autumn, and new leaves regrow in the spring. In a sense, we have similar seasons in our lives. Our emotions, thoughts, and core self are all such an important part of health that a number of years ago I started a program at the Center called 'The Path of Fulfillment.' It consists of workshops and meditations offered evenings and weekends to help you explore your transitions and embrace change. Sometimes depression is caused by low hormones, but it also signals that our old life is no longer working. I'd love you to explore and take any workshops that appeal to you. The teachers are wonderful, and the support for your growth is enormous.

"Let's sum up what is happening to you. You are menopausal, with low estrogen, low testosterone and low progesterone. Your thyroid is fine. Your adrenals are a bit stressed due to menopause, but they will be fine once we balance your estrogen. I want to prescribe Sweet Sleep, which is a great natural sleep remedy. Sleeping will help restore your body more quickly. It will also help lower your sugar level, which is borderline diabetic at this point. Stress raises blood sugar, and good sleep will decrease your stress. So really, your main problem is menopause. It has caused your weight gain, depression, anxiety, anger, fatigue, sleeplessness, low sex drive, and skin changes. Replacing your estrogen will cause all these symptoms to fade away. Any questions or confusion so far?"

"I am actually really okay. I feel like crying from relief, but I am also upset I waited this long to seek help. I feel like I'm too far down the rabbit hole ... for nothing."

"It's okay," I reassure her. "So many people come to me after being in menopause for twenty years. They drag themselves in here with all their hormones crashed, and we help them, too. So you are actually really on top of this. I am proud of you."

If it feels right, I frequently offer to say a small blessing to help the "magic" of the hormones work faster. As Julia and I finish our meeting, I offer this to her and she smiles widely in agreement. I place her estrogen and testosterone in her hands and close my eyes. "May these small molecules bring health, joy and harmony back to your body. May they join your own hormones and help them work better, performing all their vital functions. You deserve to be fabulous, loved and cared for, and I ask that these hormones help you return to your true sweetheart self."

At the end of my conversation with Julia, I see hope in her eyes. I offer a goodbye hug and her warm response tells me she needs to be hugged a whole lot more. Happiness and touch are integral to healing.

I can't work with a new client without feeling enormous gratitude for the life I have been given. I am flooded with the joy of helping Julia and look forward to seeing her life transform in mysterious and wonderful ways.

For thousands of years we have approached health not only as a physical problem, but also as emotional and soul journeys. In fact, our emotions and our ability to imagine a new way of being are frequently our most powerful doctors. The relationships we create can be very powerful in our health journey. Many women have expressed to me that they feel the cause of their cancer or heart attack was due to fear of, or anger with, a partner or with life in general.

At the end of our meeting, I introduce Julia to one of our Naturopathic Physicians who will inspire her to eat right. At the Center, we have worked hard on our diet plan. Julia is asked to begin consuming a nutritious plant-based protein smoothie each morning while eliminating grains (like gluten, corn and wheat), sugar and dairy. All of these foods cause inflammation of the brain, joints, intestines, and muscles—and inflammation is a root cause of many cancers, aging skin, heart disease, arthritis and dementia. One particular culprit is sugar, which coats our cells, causing cellular damage. Julia is clearly insulin resistant and borderline

> *Many women have expressed to me that they feel the cause of their cancer or heart attack was due to fear of, or anger with, a partner or with life in general.*

diabetic. The estrogen and diet I am prescribing will lower her sugar naturally and help avoid other interventions.

> *All of these foods cause inflammation of the brain, joints, intestines, and muscles—and inflammation is a root cause of many cancers, aging skin, heart disease, arthritis and dementia.*

Julia doesn't resist the food plan. She agrees there are plenty of food choices and she is excited to "clean up her body." In addition, Julia is given a parasite analysis kit to use within the next week or two. Many people have parasites, yeast and bacterial overgrowth that cause "leaky gut" and other chronic medical problems.

Julia next meets with our patient educator to discuss how to put her program all together. Everything is reviewed and explained: how to apply her creams, take her supplements, sleep more deeply, and eat and love herself back to health. She receives a follow-up call the day after her appointment and again in one and two weeks as part of the Core Program to answer any questions or make any adjustments to her program.

The following are the prescriptions Julia receives during her visit to the Center:

- Estradiol cream: one click AM and PM
- Testosterone cream: one click each AM
- Sweet Sleep: 1-2 capsules at bedtime
- Magnesium: 500 mg at bedtime
- A morning protein shake; no grains, dairy or sugar in her diet

This program is usually plenty for a patient to handle for a first visit. Slow and steady usually proves to be a better remedy than overloading a patient at the start.

We call Julia in two weeks to check on her, and she reports feeling happier. She has her routine down and her sleep is not quite as fitful. She hasn't had a panic attack since our first appointment and feels she is "nicer and more patient." She hasn't lost any weight yet, but once the body is calmer and less stressed the weight will naturally begin to come off. We increase her estrogen to two clicks twice a day and remind her to get her blood drawn in three weeks.

After six weeks, Julia returns for her second consultation with me, smiling in greeting.

"Oh, Prudence!" she exclaims, "I feel so much better! I know we are just beginning, but it's happening. I feel my body waking up." I hear relief in her voice.

After reviewing and explaining her new lab values, it is clear the program is working. She describes herself as feeling 30 percent less tired, but she's still waking up some in the middle of the night. I add five milligrams of melatonin to her night routine to improve her sleep and explain that melatonin also helps prevent breast cancer and dementia. The estrogen calmed her panic and moods quite a bit, but she still feels nervous. I raise her estrogen to three clicks twice a day. I instruct her to go to four clicks morning and night if her menopausal symptoms are still present after a month.

I add progesterone to Julia's regimen and explain how to "cycle" the drops each two weeks—taking drops from the first to the fifteenth of each month, and not taking them from the sixteenth through the thirty-first. In a few months we might add a bit of rhythmicity to her cycle to mimic a natural menstrual cycle. I do this by peaking her estrogen on days fourteen and fifteen of each month and her progesterone on days twenty-one and twenty-two of the month. I explain that she might resume having periods as her body returns to a balanced state. Most women in Julia's condition consider this a small price to pay for all the benefits.

The testosterone cream I prescribed has moderately raised her level, but her libido hasn't improved yet. She describes feeling less angry with her husband, though. I double her clicks of testosterone and suggest she use some Dream Cream every night. "Rub it into your clitoris and inner labial area after your shower," I tell her. "It will bring more blood to your clitoris and help you feel sexier and also have faster orgasms." In case she doesn't know how important nipple stimulation is for desire and orgasms, I suggested a great Tantric book for her to read.

Next, Julia sees one of our Naturopathic Physicians. Her stool analysis is free of parasites, even though she is craving sugar badly. Julia's detox is started, and she is asked to keep a food journal. She decides to add on weekly coaching sessions to help her stay on track with her diet and exercise. Not all clients need mentoring, but having one sure helps in achieving health and life goals.

In business, the most successful CEOs and entrepreneurs are coached. I personally have two weekly mentoring sessions with Doron Libshtein, and the sessions give me great clarity on where I am headed and what needs to be done to get there. I love mentoring! In fact, for ten years I kept telling myself I wanted to write a book. Now, because of being mentored, I have written two books in six months. It feels wonderful!

> *I personally have two weekly mentoring sessions with Doron Libshtein, and the sessions give me great clarity on where I am headed and what needs to be done to get there.*

I see Julia in two more moths for her third session and I hardly recognize her. She is beaming and has lost fifteen pounds. Her skin is moist and much more youthful, and she describes herself as having 90 percent of the energy levels she felt at thirty-five. She followed the food plan we gave her, and it shows. Her muscle mass has improved and she has enough energy to jump on the trampoline for fifteen minutes a day. Her libido has really improved, but her marriage hasn't improved to the point that she wants to have a physical relationship yet. They have begun couples counseling to address their issues. She expresses her desire to be a real partner with her husband, but she is unwilling to continue being abused verbally. I have many resources to offer struggling couples and suggest they might receive benefits from a Landmark Worldwide seminar, a powerful, transformational program my former husband and I took part in. I also suggest she check out Ger Lyons' (gerlyons.net) workshops. Ger leads cathartic Core and Cellular Transformation groups resulting in rapid change and healing. Finally, I suggest Doron Libshtein's new book, *Walk Your Path,* to help her better know herself. After all, knowing yourself and knowing your true path is the basis of forming the best relationship—with yourself and others.

Julia's situation is one I see numerous times each day. Menopause happens to all women, and we need real strategies to maintain our health and vitality. I think about my own journey of female hormonal challenges: PMS, miscarriages, pregnancies, and perimenopause. I remember when I was pregnant with my third child at age forty. What joy to finally have a successful pregnancy after two consecutive miscarriages! However, after Conrad's birth, I started having strange heat intolerances. At first I would wake up at night sweating, but then I started sweating during the day too. And I felt so tired! I also couldn't understand why I was feeling down, since I am rarely less than optimistic.

You would expect a hormone expert who has handled thousands of such cases to immediately diagnose her own hormone imbalances and to begin treatment—but somehow I missed the problem. Maybe I was too busy with the new baby and my practice, or maybe I was just trying to be brave. However, after several months when the hot flashes and other symptoms didn't go away, diagnoses started popping up in my head. I considered lymphoma, tumors, and even AIDS. Twenty years before I had stuck myself with a needle in surgery, and even though my tests were negative for years, I worried I might have contracted hepatitis from that needle stick. I am not a hypochondriac, but I confess that in my own mind I had myself quite sick and almost buried. After I got up the nerve to check my blood, the diagnosis was quite simple. I was experiencing perimenopause with all the classic symptoms, and also low thyroid due to my recent delivery. But I certainly had none of the dreaded diseases I had imagined.

As I aged, I raised my bioidentical hormone levels to keep them in the youthful range.

Relieved but a bit shaken, I started myself on a bit of bioidentical estrogen. The hot flashes immediately stopped. I added a small amount of testosterone and my confidence and muscle mass started to rebuild. I began the thyroid T3-T4 combination I use with clients, and felt much more energetic and not at all depressed. I am fortunate to have stopped the whole process quickly and easily. As I aged, my bioidentical hormones were raised to maintain youthful levels. Because of this, I have never experienced symptoms or the decline associated with menopause. I really am a firm believer in preventing harmful processes such as those associated with menopause which deplete our bones, brain, and confidence, while increasing heart disease and other diseases of aging. Thank God for bioidentical hormones!

> *Truly, we are all in this together. We are not alone.*

The lesson I learned from my experience is that if I didn't recognize my own diagnosis with all the knowledge I have, how could I expect a client to see herself accurately? Especially if she is quite young, it would be very easy to miss the diagnosis, like I did. I have compassion for all women struggling with these symptoms, and especially for women who try to muscle through their symptoms like I did. Truly, we are all in this together. We are not alone.

I was touched to receive a letter Julia wrote four months later. With her permission, I include it.

Dear Prudence,

I can't wait two months until my next appointment to tell you my good news! I am a new person, and more healthy than I was before I had my babies. I am exercising almost every day, have lost another ten pounds, sleep like a baby, and truly feel happy. Larry and I turned our relationship around and are making love like newlyweds. I don't know when I have felt this good or happy. I am so grateful. My whole life has changed, and all the work I did on eating well has also changed my life, Larry's life, my kids, and then my sisters and their kids' lives. It's like a snowball. I am now the go-to person for menopause and feel it is part of what I was sent here to do. I have a blog with tons of people joining. You wouldn't believe how many people ask me for advice and help. I love my life.

I have referred a number of people to your Center, including my sister and my best friend. They both have appointments, and I know you can help them like you did me. They are pretty desperate too. Truly, Prudence, thank you.

See you in two months. You won't believe it's me.

Love,

Julia

After reading Julia's letter, I sit back and allow myself to feel the vitality and new life coming through her letter. The real Julia was finally back and joyfully helping others. That's how it works: we are helped, and then we help others. Reading letters like Julia's causes gratitude to well up in me. I have been given such a privileged life with the knowledge I have and the opportunity to help so many people. In moments like this one, I feel true joy.

Takeaway:

Menopause occurs when the ovaries stop producing estrogen, generally around age forty-four to forty-nine. This impacts all hormonal systems and frequently results in adrenal deficiency, loss of thyroid hormones, and insulin/sugar problems. It causes havoc in the body, giving rise to most of the chronic diseases of aging, including: heart attacks, diabetes, Alzheimer's, neurodegenerative decline, cancer, osteoporosis, digestive problems, high cholesterol, high blood pressure, autoimmune diseases and inflammatory illnesses. Please avoid these dangerous conditions by balancing your hormonal software.

Healthy hormonal balance does not cause cancer. Imbalanced hormones, toxicity, poor lifestyle choices and loss of enzymes do.

Symptoms of menopause:

Fatigue, inability to fall asleep, awakening through the night, hot flashes, night sweats, depression, foggy brain, irritability, anger, weight gain, muscle loss, low sex drive, lack of orgasms, aging skin, a pounding heart, and loss of charisma and energy.

My prescription for menopause:

- Bioidentical hormones to replace any deficient hormones

- If prescriptions are not available, use Feminine Radiance (Body Software): 1-2 capsules twice daily.

- Super Adrenal (Body Software) for energy: 1-2 capsules each morning

- Bliss (Body Software): 1-2 capsules each morning for depression, irritability and anxiety

- Iodine/Biodine to support the thyroid gland: 1 capsule daily

- Sweet Sleep (Body Software): 1-2 capsules for sleep disturbances

- Magnesium: about 500 mg at bedtime for a deeper sleep

Chapter 2

Prudence and the Pill

I meet Mariuma at a fund raiser for her Shanti House residences, and experience instant love. The mission of this dear woman is to help homeless, desperate adolescents regain their lives. Mariuma started her first residential house in Israel thirty years ago and now has two Shanti residences that have housed, educated, fed and saved more than 35,000 homeless kids from many ethnic backgrounds.

"Prudence," the enthusiastic and forthright woman beams when I approach. "You're a doctor, right? I hear you do things differently, and one of my daughters, Shlomit, is suffering so much. She is just a kid and has already seen a number of other doctors who don't seem to have a clue what is wrong with her. She just moved to LA. Is there any way you might help her?"

I promise to do whatever I can and ask that Shlomit call the Center to have her blood drawn.

Shlomit arrives at the office one week later. She has dark, curly hair, a sweet smile and a joyous feeling about her. I begin our appointment by asking her to describe how she is feeling.

"Prudence, I feel terrible and haven't felt well for more than three years. I am tired—actually, I'm exhausted. And I haven't had my periods for months on end. When I do, they last twenty days. I'm miserable with awful headaches. They are like migraines, and I can't leave the house. I guess I'm depressed too, and I have gained more than ten pounds. I just moved here from New York. I'm an actress but I feel I just can't do this anymore because I'm too tired. And I have such a good boyfriend, but no sex drive at all. I've paid so much money to try to find out what has happened to me, but nothing has been uncovered. They tell me I am completely 'normal.'" Her voice rises to a slight wail of despair. "But I'm *not* normal. Something is really wrong."

This delicate girl is so dear. I check her charts and note that she is on the pill. I inquire how long she has been taking it.

"About three-and-a-half years. I was given the pill because of bad cramps."

I touch her hand. "Shlomit, by any chance did your symptoms begin after you started taking the pill?"

Shock registers on her face. "Well, maybe … I'd have to think about it." She furrows her brow and becomes silent. "Yes, actually, they did seem to begin shortly after I started the pill. But I mentioned that to my first doctor and he told me there was no correlation. Do you think the pill could have caused this?"

One glance at her blood levels chart confirms that this is true. Her estradiol levels are extremely low!

"Shlomit, I think the pill is to blame for many or perhaps all of your symptoms." I open her new patient notebook and show her the results of her blood work. "Your estrogen level is only fifteen, when two hundred is healthy for your age. Your symptoms are actually quite typical of women taking the pill; they also have low estrogen levels and many of the same symptoms you have. Your testosterone level is also low—it's twenty when it should be two to three times higher for a good sex drive. Many women tell me their sex drive is low while on the pill. Your low sex drive, fatigue and weight gain—and most likely your headaches—are all caused by the pill."

Shlomit's eyes widen. "You mean my estrogen level is fifteen? Fifteen?! Am I a man with those levels?"

> Your low sex drive, fatigue and weight gain—and most likely your headaches—are all caused by the pill.

I look at the incredibly beautiful girl and can't suppress a laugh. "If you're a man, the whole male species is going to have a whole lot to live up to. It's only the pill doing this to your body. I have measured hundreds of young women's hormones on the pill, and your low estrogen level, which is typical of a sixty-year-old woman, is what happens to most pill users."

"I can't believe this," Shlomit's dark eyes reflect her disbelief. "You mean the pill has caused all these years of illness? That's awful! No doctor has so much as raised even a single question about this."

"I know, Shlomit. It is shocking and really awful. There are millions of girls and women on the pill, yet it is rarely identified as the cause of so many symptoms. Low estrogen and testosterone, which are caused by the pill, create lots of problems for women. I see a typical downward spiral with these patients. First they get depressed due to their low estrogen level, so they are prescribed an antidepressant. Then they don't have a sex drive due to the antidepressant as well as the low estrogen *and* testosterone levels. They gain weight, which causes more depression, and then they gain more weight due to their loss of muscle mass. A menopausal woman will gain thirty or forty pounds due to her loss of estrogen, and so can pill users. Attention deficit problems, including ADHD are also caused by the pill. The brain needs estrogen to function. Memory is poor without it, and specifically the recall of nouns."

A menopausal woman will gain thirty or forty pounds due to her loss of estrogen, and so can pill users.

"Oh, my God, I can't remember my acting lines nearly as well as I could a few years ago, and one of the doctors wanted to give me Adderall to help me concentrate better. He said I had ADHD, but I refused to take the drug."

"Thank goodness you didn't; it's just a Band-Aid solution. Instead, let's get to the root of your problem, which is the pill. We'll take you off it and let your hormone levels recover. If a diseased tree has leaves that are turning brown and falling off, the answer is not to paint the leaves! But that's what these other solutions are equivalent to."

Shlomit's face registers her relief. "I agree. I was considering diet pills, because it's terrible for my career to be up ten pounds—but antidepressants, Adderall, diet pills? That's crazy! My mother lives a natural lifestyle, and I aim for that too. But I was feeling so desperate."

"Shlomit, the pill was created in the mid-1950s and it liberated women in many ways, but we didn't have a clue about hormones. The worst thing is that a significant number of women never regain healthy hormone levels after taking the pill. But that's not going to happen to you if we can get you off the pill right away."

Shlomit looks at me with such sadness, her shoulders collapsed. "Of course I'll come off. I'm just so upset I have been doing this to myself. Can I come off today?"

> *The pill was created in the mid-1950s and it liberated women in many ways, but we didn't have a clue about hormones.*

"Absolutely. Just stop the pack, but I'm concerned that you may initially feel a bit worse before your own hormones return to proper levels. I'll prescribe a small amount of bioidentical estrogen cream to help with the transition for the next few months. My nurses will show you how to use the cream. But Shlomit, there is another test that was a bit abnormal. It's your Thyroflex score."

Her face expresses concern. "My what?"

"It's the reflex test we did on your arm with the little hammer. It shows that your reflexes are quite slow, which in 95 percent of cases means you have low thyroid."

Shlomit looks puzzled. "Well, I saw all those other doctors and no one mentioned my thyroid—but I'll do whatever you think I need to do!" Her smile lights up the room.

I smile at her youthful and enchanting enthusiasm. "Well, let's go slowly to see if your thyroid recovers. Low thyroid can be associated with birth control pill use but hopefully, as the pill leaves your body, your thyroid gland will work better. Let's begin with a natural iodine supplement to help your thyroid gland function more effectively. I want you to recover as quickly as possible. Shall we say a little blessing to make this possible?"

Shlomit is tearful, overcome by the possibility of feeling well again, and nods her head.

I close my eyes and go inward. "May the pill leave your body like a river plummeting down a steep mountain, filling you with robust health. May your brain wake up and feel the joy of each moment, and your body become strong and loving again, returning you to your natural joyful self."

After a brief silence, Shlomit opens her eyes and I see new strength and resolve in them. "It is happening, Prudence. I feel it, and I know I'll be better, just like you said."

"Yes you will, dear one, yes you will." I know that all change, both physical and emotional, starts with believing it will happen. When we can see, feel, touch and literally taste the change we need, it is like rocket fuel for the outcome to manifest.

"Do you have any questions? Do you understand what we need to do?"

"A-1 clear. It's gonna happen and I'm going to help it happen."

"You won't be alone. We'll call you three or four times to see how you're feeling, and don't hesitate to call us if you have questions." We hug and I walk her to our Naturopathic doctor to discuss her diet.

After two weeks, Shlomit is using a bit of her estrogen cream and feels slightly better, but nothing dramatic. I tell her to use a bit more and suggest waiting a few more months to give her body a chance to recover.

On my next trip to Israel, I see her mother Mariuma, who throws her arms around me. "You have saved my daughter! She is back to her normal self and feels wonderful. You don't know how awful this has been to have her so ill." Relief floods through me, because I haven't heard from Shlomit recently.

A week later, I am filled with anticipation when I look at my schedule and see her name. I greet her warmly, both of us smiling widely.

"I am wonderful!" she exclaims as she sits down. "I had a regular period without cramps for a normal number of days. I am so happy … and look at me! I've lost five pounds. I can't believe it. I kept gaining before. No headaches either. Really, I feel great, although I'm still a bit tired."

I look at Shlomit's most recent blood tests and see that her estrogen and testosterone levels are rapidly coming back to normal. She is one of the lucky ones who is recovering quickly! However, her Thyroflex test hasn't improved with the iodine I prescribed, which confirms Shlomit has low thyroid. At my suggestion she opts to try a small amount of thyroid hormone. Two weeks later I receive an email from her:

> Dear Prudence,
>
> The little bit of thyroid you gave me helped so much, and so did coming off the pill. Every day I feel stronger and more like myself. I am almost totally "back" again. I am so relieved not to be depressed anymore. My question is this: can I take a bit more thyroid? My memory is much better, but I am still having a problem memorizing long lines. I think the thyroid is helping with that. But really, I am great. All those low sex drive symptoms are completely gone and I am getting along great with my boyfriend. Truly, I am a completely new person.
>
> If you ever want to dine at the restaurant where I am working, I will get you in even though it usually takes weeks to get a reservation.
>
> See you soon.
>
> Love,
>
> Shlomit

I agree with Shlomit that she needs a bit more thyroid, so we raise her dose one half grain. I also take her up on her kind offer. When my guests and I arrive at the restaurant a few weeks later, we are greeted by an ebullient and outgoing beauty filled with energy and life. She is also quite startlingly thin. "This is the way I used to be," she assures me. She throws her arms around me then my guests—and they all fall in love with her, just as I did.

Three months later Shlomit's blood tests are back to normal and so is her Thyroflex exam. She is one of the fortunate ones, because many patients require more time to get their hormone levels back in order.

Soon after, another young woman comes in to discuss hormone levels with me. Susan is twenty-one years old and one of the sweetest young women I know—and I know her well because she is the beloved girlfriend of one of my sons.

Susan jumps right in. "I don't know why I feel so irritable and tired. This isn't like me at all. And I'm getting PMS, which makes me feel a bit down. I'm not depressed, but I'm just not myself. That son of yours keeps telling me to see you, so here I am."

Susan relates that her sleep also is off. In addition, though she rides bikes, walks, and is always active, her muscles are kind of soft and she is gaining weight. I have been hoping for this opportunity to speak to her, because my son has told me she is on the pill—and he of course knows my bias against it.

"Tell me more," I encourage her.

"I just don't feel happy like I normally do. And I'm waking up a lot in the night. My muscles ache more after exercising, and I feel kind of old. I don't know. It's just these vague feelings of being 'off.'"

"Let's look at your hormones, Susan. Ideal estrogen levels are 150, maybe even 200. Your level is 20. Below 30 is menopausal."

She covers her mouth in a gasp and grabs my arm. "So I can't have children?" Her eyes are stricken.

I reach out quickly, touching her hand. "No, no ... of course you can have kids. I am so sorry I scared you. I only meant to convey that the pill has suppressed your hormone levels and put you into a temporary menopause. That's why you're feeling so poorly. Considering your levels, you're actually doing really well, but these low levels aren't good for you. Would you like to come off the pill?"

> *Ideal estrogen levels are 150, maybe even 200. Your level is 20. Below 30 is menopausal.*

"Actually, I would. I have been thinking of using the IUD and have read everything about it. What do you think? I don't want to get pregnant yet."

"The IUD is a good choice," I respond, "but your periods will be heavier and you might have more cramps. The real concern is whether an IUD could cause infertility problems. The Copper T Paraguard Company suggests that IUDs shouldn't be used by young women who haven't had babies, but those restrictions are lessening in the medical community. I actually feel there are fewer fertility problems with an IUD than with taking the pill."

"I need something better than condoms or a diaphragm, and I understand the infertility problem is more common when a woman is not monogamous. But that's not a concern for me."

I smile with love. "It's very important to be sure you don't have any STDs or anything before the IUD is inserted. As long as you use condoms with any future partners and check them for STDs, I think you are pretty safe. We never know about our fertility, but I feel this is safer than the birth control pill. And we can measure your hormones to make sure you're recovering from the pill."

Susan calls me a few days later. She's had the IUD inserted at UCLA where she works and is in agony, sobbing and scared. "I have terrible cramps and awful pain. I feel like I'm having a child or something. I'm shaking and feel like vomiting; it is so bad, Prudence."

We discuss how the IUD can cause cramps for a few weeks after being placed. I recommend Advil and a hot water bottle or heating pad for relief. As we talk, Susan tells me how angry she feels.

> *I actually feel there are fewer fertility problems with an IUD than with taking the pill.*

I address one of her unspoken fears. "First of all, you *will* be able to get pregnant when you want to. I'm sure of that. This hasn't caused damage to your reproductive system."

She stops crying. "Really? You don't think I have hurt myself?"

"No, this kind of pain can happen and the doctor should have warned you."

"I can't believe they didn't tell me it might hurt like this. I can't work and am really not well. They need to learn how to treat patients!"

I reassure her that many women have a few tough weeks after IUD insertion. Knowing this calms Susan. Over the next few weeks her pain lessens, though it does continue off and on for several weeks before abating altogether.

A few months later, Susan tells me how glad she is to be off the pill. "Oh, my God, I didn't even know how bad I was feeling. I am happy; I don't feel irritated, and I've lost five pounds—so I feel much more like my old self. And even though I have always been crazy about your son, I'm even crazier about him now. I feel in better contact with my emotions. Really, I'm sorry I was on the pill for four years. I'm telling all my girlfriends to come off their pills. It is just amazing to feel so good."

Bingo! Another soldier against the pill!

I think back to my own history with the birth control pill. I was at UC Santa Cruz in my first year of college and involved with my first serious boyfriend. We decided we needed birth control and felt the pill would be a good option. I made an appointment with a doctor for my first pap smear so I could get a prescription. I was a bit apprehensive already, but it was worse than what I had imagined. I left feeling horrible about the whole process. When I decided to be a gynecologist, it was this experience that made me vow I would never, ever approach a woman like I had been approached. That experience made me realize how important it was to collaborate with my patients and empower them with their own health.

> *When I decided to be a gynecologist, it was this experience that made me vow I would never, ever approach a woman like I had been approached.*

After that exam, I began using the pill but soon started feeling bloated and less happy than usual. At first, I attributed it to being a bit homesick for Europe, but I also began feeling anxious, insecure, and irritated with my boyfriend. My sex drive was lower than usual, and as the months passed I felt more tired and became less outgoing. This went on for a year until I returned to France to continue studying at the University of Toulouse. When my new French boyfriend realized I was on the pill, he suggested I stop taking it. When I did, the positive changes were almost immediate. My body felt more lithe and my brain function improved. I was happier and also regained my outgoing and lively personality.

In spite of that misadventure, I didn't really understand how much the pill affected a woman's hormones. As a young gynecologist, I prescribed the pill to hundreds of patients. In all my training there had never been any discussion of the pill causing any of the symptoms I experienced while on the pill. It wasn't until I was in private practice for a few years that I began to understand what the pill was doing to my patients. Those women frequently complained of excessive fatigue, depression, lack of sexual desire and foggy brain function. I began measuring my pill patients' estrogen levels and was shocked to find their levels similar to my much older menopausal patients.

After taking hundreds of patients off the pill over many years, I came to understand that the birth control pill actually created a hormonal menopause. I saw firsthand the profound hormonal imbalances, with a significant number of patients taking years to recover. I was dismayed that some of my patients actually never fully recovered, needing to use small amounts of bioidentical hormones to maintain their health.

What is the bottom line? There are better and safer methods to prevent pregnancy. Too many women complain of debilitating symptoms with pill use. In addition, there is a 10 percent reported increase in breast cancer, more cervical problems, increased deep vein clots, and in my experience, much more depression, weight gain, ADHD, headaches, muscle and joint pain, sexual dysfunction, fertility problems, and loss of self-confidence. When my patients request the pill, I always urge them to consider other options.

> *There are better and safer methods to prevent pregnancy. Too many women complain of debilitating symptoms with pill use.*

When looking at other choices, keep in mind that each woman responds individually. Unfortunately, the patch, ring, and Depo Provera shot are all similar to the birth control pill, resulting in similar problems. My recommendation for helping women avoid pregnancy while remaining sexy and healthy is to use condoms, the diaphragm, withdrawal, or the Paraguard IUD. My main objective is to avoid disturbing a woman's own hormone production, but if other contraceptive methods are declined, bioidentical hormones used as a birth control method are an option. While the bioidentical hormones will stop ovulation just like the birth control pill does, they will not deprive a woman's body of the hormones it needs.

Takeaway:

The birth control pill decreases the body's natural hormonal balance of estrogen, testosterone and progesterone. When I analyze the hormones of a woman on the pill, her levels look like a sixty-year-old's hormones, with the exception of her FSH being low.

My prescription for pill users:

- Discontinue the pill and begin a non hormonal method of birth control such as condoms, Paraguard IUD or the diaphragm

- Bliss (Body Software): 1-2 capsules per day to help with any depression arising from pill use

- Brilliant Brain (Body Software): 2 capsules per day to help the brain recover from the pill

- Chasteberry (Vitex) 500mg: take 1 capsule AM and PM for several months to help rebalance your estrogen levels. You may stop once your periods resume regularly.

- Eat a healthy diet. Sleep 8 hours per night.

- I love the WellBe to help identify and reduce stress.

Chapter 3

Perimenopause and PMS Blues—Get Me Out of Here!

I greet my new patient, Michelle, who came from San Diego, with her boyfriend. Her beautiful blue eyes look anxious and the puffiness beneath them tells me she's tired. I usher them into my consultation room and as I hug Michelle, I realize she is freezing cold! Andrew is tanned and fit, and I pick up an accent as he greets me.

"You're not English, and not Australian ... are you from New Zealand?" I ask.

"No," he replies, chuckling and flashing me a wide, enchanting smile. "I'm from South Africa."

Michelle is equally charming. "I've waited so long to see you, and I'm so happy to finally be here!"

My assistant brings them some tea and we begin our conversation. "Michelle, tell me everything! I am eager to help."

"Well, I began experiencing PMS about two years after the birth of my last child. I'm forty-five now, so I was about thirty-eight at the time. I started having hot flashes and felt really depressed before my period. I thought I was in perimenopause and saw a doctor who put me on natural progesterone. He didn't test my levels before prescribing it, and it felt like a generic approach to my problem. I wondered whether I should be taking something that was tailored to my needs. I felt a tiny bit better, but not enough to continue, so I stopped the hormones a year later. Since then I have continued to struggle with terrible PMS and it's harder to deal with, given all the stress I'm under."

I look at her closely. "Michelle, I totally agree. Stress really does make everything worse. It causes so much of our body chemistry to become imbalanced. Can you tell me what's causing the stress?"

> *He didn't test my levels before prescribing estrogen or anything though, and it felt like a generic approach to my problem.*

"Well, the stress is better now, but it doesn't help that my twenty-three-year-old son is a heroin addict and almost died several times."

"In fact, he did die," Andrew chimes in. "He was clinically flat-line, but they brought him back. Throughout all this Michelle has been amazing—very centered and loving."

Michelle continues. "He's better now and in a recovery facility in Oregon, but at one point I had to let him go and he was homeless on the street. It started with Oxycontin . . ."

I reach out to touch her hand. "I am so happy he is in a secure place now. There's really no greater pain than being helpless in the face of our children's pain."

"My older daughter is autistic. She has Asperger's Syndrome, and that's been challenging. She's a good student now but it took so many interventions." Michelle lets out a deep sigh.

"I fully understand. My nephew has Asperger's Syndrome too, so I have witnessed my sister's stress while raising him. I'm so happy your daughter is doing better now—people with Asperger's are unique, and so smart. But with all this stress, you haven't been able to concentrate much on yourself, have you?"

"No, not at all." Michelle hangs her head. "And my PMS is just awful. I'm really wicked before my period. Poor Andrew. He is such a good man and I'm terrible to him!"

Andrew interjects. "Really, she's great except for ten days before her period. Then she's really tired and a different person. It's like a light goes out. I have to be really careful around that time or I can get in a lot of trouble!"

I look at Andrew with sympathy. "I understand. It's like there's a line drawn in the sand, and you can't cross it even a tiny bit at PMS time or it's off with your head."

"Well, let me tell you, I can't even get anywhere near that line!" He laughs in such a good-natured way that I wish he could give other men lessons. "I keep track of her periods and know exactly when it's danger time." He whips out his phone and shows me his calendar.

"Michelle," I ask, "is it okay for Andrew to comment on your health? Sometimes it can feel a bit like criticism."

"No, no … it's absolutely okay. He's my best friend. We talk about everything."

"Good, Michelle, you deserve a knight in your court. How long have you been together?"

"It's been about two-and-a-half years now."

"And they have been such good years," Andrew adds. "Michelle is amazing at how she stays so calm and on top of everything."

Michelle smiles and shakes her head in a lovely, sensual manner.

"How is your sex drive?" I ask her.

Andrew responds for her. "She is always ready. It's great. If anything, my drive is low."

"Can we check his levels?" Michelle asks.

"Of course we can. I take care of many young men with low testosterone due to exhaustion and stress. How old are you now, Andrew?"

Andrew is forty-four, and as we talk I recognize that many of his symptoms pertain to low testosterone. At his request I give him a lab slip so we can work on balancing

> *Some of my most joyful moments as a doctor happen when couples reunite in sensual happiness and bliss.*

his hormones too. Some of my most joyful moments as a doctor happen when couples reunite in sensual happiness and bliss. A happy couple is an inspiration to the world. Michelle and Andrew are exemplary of a supportive and loving relationship. Even though Andrew does well with his beloved's PMS, I have seen other men leave their relationships in despair over how they are treated.

I encourage Michelle to tell me more about her PMS.

"The ten days before my period are really bad. I have headaches and am so tired that I just lie on the couch and cry. And I feel so angry! Andrew can't do anything right. I yell at him and I fight over nothing. I actually feel sick. Really, Prudence, it's awful."

"But she's great the rest of the time," Andrew adds with a smile. "Absolutely perfect!"

"It that true, Michelle? Or do you feel a bit tired the whole month, so that you need to muscle through the first two weeks of your cycle and kind of fake it?" I'm asking because I'm beginning to understand that she is a very strong person.

"You're right. I do hide some of the fatigue I am feeling all month long, but it's much worse at PMS time."

"Any weight gain? Sugar cravings, cramps or bloating?"

"Absolutely," Michelle responds. "I definitely get bloated—I think my puffy eyes are due to that. I also get terrible cramps. I have to lie in bed with a heating pad. I can't move for a few days."

I open Michelle's new patient notebook like a general heading into battle. "Okay, we have work to do and problems to solve, so let's look at your hormone levels. Do you see your FSH? The level is six. Ideal levels of this brain hormone are two to five. I consider even a slight elevation such as your level to be the first signs of perimenopause. This means you're barely entering into perimenopause, which causes fatigue and worsens PMS. Do you see how your estrogen levels are a little low? This is an important finding, because low estrogen is the cause of most PMS symptoms. It can happen at any time in a woman's life—not just in perimenopause—but it usually worsens as a woman ages and begins to lose her estrogen. I have absolutely no doubt that your PMS is mainly due to your cyclical low estrogen.

"PMS is also caused by thyroid imbalances. Your thyroid levels are low, which is why you are tired all month and not just before your period. Most doctors wouldn't diagnose you as having low thyroid, if they approached your diagnosis in a traditional manner. This condition is missed frequently. But your thyroid hormones are below the ideal range and your Thyroflex score is elevated. This FDA-approved reflex test is 90 to 95 percent accurate in diagnosing thyroid conditions; it's actually much more accurate than blood work. Your score is very high, meaning you have low thyroid, which contributes to your PMS. Your adrenals look really great." I turn the chart toward her. "See how strong your levels are? I am surprised they are so healthy with everything you are dealing with. Your D3 is low at nineteen—it should be between sixty-five and one hundred. Low D3 definitely contributes to the depression women feel with PMS."

"Wow, there are a lot of things wrong, aren't there?" Michelle notes with relief. "That means we can fix them ... doesn't it?"

"Michelle, I predict it will be rather easy to make your PMS go away." I smile at both of them. "You recognized you needed help before going into menopause which makes everything easier. Let's discuss how to fix this. I'd like you to begin the lowest dose of estrogen cream all month long, and use a bit more during your ten days of PMS to balance you out. I'd also like to prescribe the smallest dose of natural thyroid and put you on some iodine to see if that will help. You might not need thyroid forever if your thyroid gland heals. Does this make sense to you?"

Both Michelle and Andrew seem to understand everything perfectly. Michelle told me initially that she had read all of Suzanne Somers' books, which makes our consult very easy for me. I love educated patients!

"You had your nutritional consult before seeing me and I see you were prescribed a gluten-free diet to help heal your thyroid. I'm happy you'll also have protein shakes, some healthy Evening Oil of Primrose, and our Feminine Radiance supplement to help with PMS. This is all great!"

Andrew jumps in once more. "The nutritionist said her diet is incredible—organic, with lots of greens."

"I can tell. She's beautiful!" (It is always so much easier when patients are already eating a good diet.) "I have a suggestion concerning your ongoing stress levels. We have a wearable bracelet in the store called the WellBe that monitors your stress. When it tips into the danger level you receive a message and a solution to lower the stress. The suggestion might be a quick breathing exercise, music, or a short meditation. It depends upon which solution interrupts stress the fastest for you. Does that sound like something that would interest you?"

"I always wanted to meditate," Michelle replies and smiles. "Do you have someone who can teach me how? I think it would be really good for me, because even though I am managing and Andrew is a real prince, I need help during all these crises. I feel stress is aging me."

I tell her we have meditation classes every Wednesday night at the Center with wonderful teachers and private lessons with Anil Chandwani. I also recommend mentorschannel.com, which has the largest meditation library available online. Our chairman, Doron Libshtein, is the founder, bringing meditation to millions of people worldwide.

After two weeks Michelle lets me know she definitely has more energy. She hasn't reached her PMS time yet, but she feels a great deal of optimism. She is meditating and loving it. She also has made plans to participate in some of the Center's workshops next month.

Both Michelle and Andrew return six weeks after her initial appointment. Andrew had his blood drawn a few weeks ago, so we'll be discussing solutions for both of them.

Michelle jumps right in. "My PMS is so much better. Really, by at least 50 percent. I didn't cry this month. I still had cramps, but they were so much better. I am not nearly as tired as I used to be, and it is kind of amazing that I have a third of my life back!"

"I'm not giving up my PMS calendar yet," Andrew confesses with a chuckle, "but at least I wasn't counting the days until it was over. She really is much better. It is remarkable."

"That is fantastic!" I reach out to touch each of them on the hand and smile as I feel the energy flow among us. Touch is one of the most healing forms of therapy available.

"Michelle, you had your blood drawn a week before your cycle, giving us an accurate progesterone level—and your level is perfect."

When I first started my practice I tried to treat PMS with progesterone, but more often than not it didn't help patients and even made them worse. I point to her estradiol number. "See how your number is still a bit low a week before your period is due? It's better than last time, but during your ten days of PMS, let's raise your estrogen cream to three clicks in the morning and three in the evening. If you start having headaches, one dose added midday should resolve it. I predict you'll feel only the most minor symptoms of PMS, or none at all."

> *I predict you'll feel only the most minor symptoms of PMS or none at all.*

"I can't believe it, but my headaches are completely gone," Michelle exclaims.

"Good, and your thyroid looks great. Let's add magnesium at bedtime to help with the cramps and also a bit of omega 3 oil each morning. Your anti-inflammatory diet will also help with the cramps."

"I find that if I begin meditating when I have cramps, they almost go away. I love it, and I have taught my kids how to meditate too." Michelle's smile makes her glow. "My older son meditates regularly now."

"I do it every day, too," Andrew chimes in. "Well, sometimes I get too busy, but really, this is connecting Michelle and me in a deeper way. Our lovemaking is going through the roof."

I glance at his chart. His testosterone level is only 355 (ideal is 800 plus). I smile, because I know that they will reach a roof above the roof they're going through once he is balanced. I love helping such genuinely good people. One for the home team!

After I help Andrew balance his hormones our session is finished and they both see our Naturopathic doctor to discuss Michelle's stool tests—she has a parasite and will need treatment.

> *I love helping such genuinely good people. One for the home team!*

When Andrew comes for his six-week follow up, Michelle can't wait to update me—in fact, the words just pour out of her. "It's a miracle. No PMS. NONE! Really, I see how much I was actually trying to ignore feeling bad. I was ridiculously brave. I don't have to expend all that effort now. I'm just fine and Andrew is amazing. I mean he is always amazing, but now he is even more so. He wants to make love so much more and is just so positive about everything. Not that he was ever negative, but he is really powerful now; he's like Superman in terms of how he approaches his work and the problems we're facing." Her voice trails off. "Oh, no! I had better let him talk! Sorry, I just couldn't help it."

Andrew is on top of the world. A highlight in his life is how his new practice of meditation has deepened his connection to himself, Michelle, and what he calls the "light of life." Moments like these are why I am a doctor—to help patients reconnect to their true potential and greatest joy. I've always known that we are energetic-spiritual beings housed in physical vessels. Addressing energetic-spiritual roots is just as important as balancing hormones. Changing your consciousness changes your biology.

I think about the hundreds and perhaps thousands of cases of PMS I've treated over the years. One sixteen-year-old girl was cutting herself during her PMS. She was given strong antidepressants to help control the cutting, but by the time I saw her she had gained seventy-five pounds from the medication and had no energy. She cried through our entire consult. I prescribed our natural mood enhancer called Bliss, small amounts of bioidentical estrogen cream during her PMS time, and a schedule to slowly decrease her antidepressants over a three-month period. I suggested a super clean diet and had her work with Priya, a talented Trilo Therapy practitioner and integrated healer, based on the work of Zen master Nissim Amon, to understand who was really in charge of her life—her heart or her mind. She got well in

> *Moments like these are why I am a doctor—to help patients reconnect to their true potential and greatest joy.*

record time, completely stopped all cutting activity, and is now in Israel studying to become a Trilo Therapy practitioner.

Another PMS success story involves my friend's daughter who became anxious and very depressed during two weeks of each monthly cycle. During those weeks she was constantly in the emergency room with stomach pains, rashes, and unrelenting headaches. She would also hide in her room for hours, refusing to come out. She couldn't concentrate, much less do her job, and her teeth would literally be chattering from fear. After months of suffering she came to me sobbing, saying she couldn't take it anymore. I finally convinced her to come off the pill and her PMS improved by about 30 percent. The Body Software Bliss supplement helped another 30 percent, and estrogen cream during her PMS weeks almost completed her physical recovery. Her healing was completed when she began meditating and going to our Path of Fulfillment workshops. After six months she became her calm and radiant self again. Her case was not a quick fix, so it required patience on her part.

I have waged my own battles with PMS. When I was eighteen years old, I remember losing a Monopoly game with my sisters. Inexplicably, I began crying in utter despair, and I think I might have even upset the board! The next day I couldn't believe I had acted like that—I was in shock. Then an hour later my period began and the light bulb went on! From that moment on I knew that women had different sides: logical, irrational, loving, rage-filled—crazy!

> *After six months, she became her calm and radiant self again. Her case was not a quick fix, so it required patience on her part.*

In my thirties my PMS took on a different flavor. I developed obsessive-compulsive behaviors a week before my period. I've always been a bit worried about dirt and germs and liked order in my environment but at PMS time I didn't want to touch door handles. I would clean the house in the most obsessive ways and would check several times to make sure I had locked the doors at night and turned off the stove. I was shocked to find that every single symptom disappeared as soon as I treated myself with small amounts of bioidentical estrogen during my PMS time; I just couldn't believe my OCD was caused by low estrogen. From that moment on I began to observe how estrogen resolved a wide variety of symptoms my patients were experiencing at PMS time: bulimic behaviors, suicidal thoughts, increased accidents and clumsiness, overspending, manic types of behaviors, lack of sexual caution, binge drinking … the list goes on and on.

> *The good news is that PMS is fixable, and the solutions are so healthy that there is no reason at all not to fix the problem immediately.*

I am here to tell you with the utmost certainty that hormones determine much of our behavior and certainly play an important role in most of our emotions. When I first realized this, I actually got a bit depressed because I had thought I was a "free, independent agent." But I also came to realize that human "software" is comprised of hormones, enzymes, healthy food, positive thoughts and balanced body chemistry, just like plants must have water and light. I saw how each of us has an amazing, unique body with its own delicate balance of software. PMS represents an upset to that balance and creates unnecessary pain and suffering. The good news is that PMS is fixable, and the solutions are so healthy that there is no reason at all not to fix the problem immediately.

Takeaway:

PMS is a common set of unpleasant symptoms that occur before the menstrual period. In 95 percent of cases, the root cause is low estrogen, although diet, sleep, stress, and nutrient deficiency all play a role. In rare cases PMS may be triggered by a progesterone deficiency, but in most cases progesterone supplementation exacerbates PMS.

Symptoms:

The symptoms of PMS are irritability, breast tenderness, bloating, hunger, headaches, depression, weight gain, sugar and alcohol cravings, hot flashes, night sweats, low libido, and obsessive behaviors.

My prescription for PMS:

- Anti-inflammatory diet
- Bioidentical estrogen cream at PMS time, if you have access to a doctor who will prescribe it
- The Body Software supplement Feminine Radiance: 1-2 capsules twice daily at PMS time
- Bliss (Body Software): 1-2 capsules per day for irritability, anxiety, and control of hunger
- Evening Primrose Oil: 1500 mg per day
- B vitamins
- Magnesium: 500-1000 mg at bedtime to help with sleep (too much causes loose stools)
- Body Software Sweet Sleep to help with insomnia: 1-2 capsules at sleep

Chapter 4

Your Thyroid Gland

Mrs. Azim has flown in from Dubai. She is well dressed in a sophisticated suit, with her hair pulled back in a stylish manner. I smile as I welcome her into my office. Her eyes meet mine with sadness, but I sense courage and a direct and open energy.

"It is such a pleasure meeting you, Mrs. Azim! Your sister told me at her last consult that you were coming to see me."

"I should have come a long time ago, but I didn't listen to my sister. She has been telling me for years about you and how well she feels … but … I don't know." Mrs. Azim drops her head. "I guess I just didn't listen. I don't know why…"

As her voice trails off, I smile with empathy. "It's not always easy with sisters. I have three and we don't always listen to each other either. That's how sisters are—we all feel we know what's best for ourselves. But you are here now, so this must be the best and right time for you to come. Tell me what's troubling you. I am truly interested in helping any way I can."

She lets out a deep breath. "Well, I haven't been feeling like myself for years. I am married to a good man, but one who is stubborn and has to have his own way. I was an interpreter before I married him, and little by little he encouraged me to give up my work. I have two boys, sixteen and twenty-three. As I got busier with them it made sense not to work. Now I regret stopping, because I don't have a life of my own anymore. My son is done with college and working with my husband in our business, and my youngest is quite independent. He doesn't need me much. I used to be very social and host dinner parties or go out with our friends. I felt quite full of energy. Now I am just so tired. I don't feel like doing much. I feel I am pretty much finished." She pauses as sadness floods her eyes. "I mean I have had a career, marriage, children; my life feels done. I did what I needed to do and now there's really nothing left for me."

> *My heart opens as I recall my own dark nights of the soul, where I questioned everything about myself.*

I look down at her hands and they are shaking. I pull my chair closer. I am talking with a woman from the Middle East where close distances are reassuring, not threatening. And she is in pain. My heart opens as I recall my own dark nights of the soul, where I questioned everything about myself. I shiver, knowing how fragile our happiness and our lives can be. "I understand," I tell her. "When one book has been written, it can feel like there is nothing more to say—sometimes for a long time. But the interesting thing is, this sorrow you are experiencing actually offers you the opportunity to really get to know who you are and what you are meant to do. You now have time and a need to know.

> *"Did you know that your emotions are almost completely dependent on your hormones?"*

I have three children, and I certainly lost track of who I was and what I needed when they were young."

"I see what you mean." She sighs. "But I have no will and certainly no energy to think about those things. I am just exhausted."

"Well, let's get you feeling well again and then later we can return to this topic of your life. Did you know that your emotions are almost completely dependent on your hormones?"

Her eyes show her surprise. "I wasn't aware of that. I have always tried to stay positive, because I know my thoughts are important in terms of causing depression."

"Absolutely right, but healthy, balanced hormones cause positive thoughts without trying so much. So, when did you start to feel badly?"

"Well, I don't really know." Mrs. Azim looks up to the ceiling. "I just started feeling a bit tired, probably from the stress of being a mother, but it didn't get better. Then I became depressed, and my doctor sent me to a psychiatrist for antidepressants. Over the years they've changed me from one medicine to another. I am currently taking Celexa, and I am certain it causes my brain to be so forgetful and fuzzy." Her eyes lock on mine and I see her fear. "I think I might even be developing dementia. I was in my car the other day and I forgot where I was going. I had to pull over and think about it. This is why I don't have great hope about the future. I don't

> *"Absolutely right, but healthy, balanced hormones cause positive thoughts without trying so much."*

know if my brain will ever recover, but I can't go on like this. I am actually afraid to go out. What if I forget where I live? I am just old and broken down."

> *I notice she has lost some of her eyebrows, especially the outer part—and this is a helpful clue in making the correct diagnosis.*

I take her hand in mine. "But Mrs. Azim, you are only forty-five! You're a young woman with another sixty years ahead of you. I promise that by the time we finish today you'll understand why you feel the way you do, and you won't feel so alone and afraid."

"You're right. I am not old." She straightens up in her chair. "But look at my hair and skin. I am drying up. And I *look* old even if I'm not. Look at my body! I have gained at least ten pounds and it is all around my middle. I am just not who I used to be."

I look at her beautiful dark hair. Yes, it's dry and the ends look a bit frayed, but it is still a crowning glory. And her face is so youthful. She could perhaps stand to lose those ten pounds, but she is really a unique beauty. I marvel at how hard we women are on ourselves and how much our feelings influence how we see the world and ourselves. I notice she has lost some of her eyebrows, especially the outer part—and this is a helpful clue in making the correct diagnosis.

"Have all these problems continued to get worse?"

"It's been ten years of slowly going downhill, little by little. The last three years have been the worst. I am really constipated, and my stomach hurts all the time. And my mind is awful, as I mentioned before."

"Well, we need to correct this right away. You have jumped out of the airplane without your parachute. Let's look at your tests together." I reach for her chart from the table beside us. "The pieces of this puzzle are right here. First, here are your thyroid hormone blood values. Do you see your TSH? When your brain needs more thyroid hormone it sends out higher TSH levels, causing your thyroid gland to release more hormones. Your TSH value is borderline high at 2.4. Also your free T3 is 2.3, which is not in the ideal range. Ideal is much higher. Based solely on your blood work, I believe your thyroid is low. The FDA-approved Thyroflex test we just did for you measures your reflexes. The test is 95 percent accurate in diagnosing thyroid disorders, and it confirms what we found in the blood work. You scored 176, and a number above 100 indicates poor thyroid function.

"Typical symptoms of low thyroid are fatigue, weight gain, depression, hair loss, dry skin, feeling cold, and constipation. It also causes muscle loss resulting in sagging skin. You have mentioned most of these symptoms, and in fact indicated thirty-seven symptoms of low thyroid on your questionnaire. I have absolutely no doubt that you have hypo (low) thyroid."

Mrs. Azim covers her mouth with her hands and stifles a gasp. "Dr. Hall, I can't believe this. I just can't believe this is the cause of my symptoms. I've gone to four different doctors over the last ten years but nobody has diagnosed this. It is really unbelievable! I am so upset. You mean this is why I am so tired and depressed? You don't think I have dementia?"

"I think your brain fog will clear right up once we resolve this. Low thyroid causes a form of dementia, but it's treatable and completely curable. And yes, I think this is surely what is causing your depression, fatigue, and most of your other symptoms. All the rest of your tests are quite normal. It's very upsetting, especially because you've wrongly been put on antidepressants. They have so many side effects, and they weren't even treating the root cause of your depression."

Almost daily, I see patients with multiple symptoms just like Mrs. Azim's. They have been diagnosed with unusual and bizarre diagnoses, or they feel they have cancer or some other terrible disease. They are so relieved to find out that a single, easily treatable condition is often behind it all. These patients are in a state of disbelief when they learn all their suffering could have been prevented.

"I am so truly sorry, Mrs. Azim. I regret that so many doctors in the medical profession diagnose strictly 'by the book.' And the 'book' is often a medical book from twenty years ago. But if a doctor isn't aware of thyroid disease being a subtle diagnosis, it can easily be missed. What I have come to understand is that so-called normal thyroid levels from blood tests don't necessarily mean those levels are ideal for one person, even though they might be fine for another. Also, most doctors use only blood work to make

> *Low thyroid causes a form of dementia, but it's treatable and completely curable.*

their diagnosis. They are not aware that blood values are only 50 to 60 percent diagnostic. Laboratories create their reference ranges from a random test group, which includes results from patients with undiagnosed hypothyroid conditions. The inclusion of that kind of patient skews the entire 'normal' range for blood values."

> *When we started studying cholesterol values from countries with very low incidences of heart disease, we realized that healthy cholesterol levels should be much lower in the 120 to 180 range, rather than our "sick population" norms.*

"This is amazing; I wish I had known this ten years ago."

I nod in agreement. "I'm so sorry it was missed."

This use of faulty values for normal reference ranges occurred years ago with cholesterol testing. I remember when a cholesterol level of 250 or even 275 was considered normal. Doctors couldn't understand why a patient would have a normal cholesterol test result and then suffer a heart attack a week later. When we started studying cholesterol values from countries with very low incidences of heart disease, we realized that healthy cholesterol levels should be much lower in the 120 to 180 range, rather than our "sick population" norms. We lowered our reference ranges, which resulted in much more effective prevention of heart disease.

"For the last ten years we have been in the middle of a hypothyroid epidemic, which has caused us to include a lot of sick thyroid values in our normal ranges. There is also an epidemic of thyroid cancer. Atomic testing, nuclear power plant disasters, a high grain diet, low iodine consumption, intestinal damage from sugar and gluten allergies, and widespread mercury, cadmium and lead toxicity have all played a part in causing this epidemic of thyroid disease. We need to detoxify our bodies of these harmful carcinogens and consume adequate amounts of iodine. But that's a lot of information. Is it too much to digest?"

"No, absolutely not." Mrs. Azim beams. "I understand, and I want to know what my body is doing and what's going on. I can't believe doctors are still using only blood values, and not even accurate ones! Doctors have been so arrogant when I asked them questions. I felt like I shouldn't even ask things. Really, I feel quite angry. I think I deserve an apology from all those doctors who tried to stop my questions, then gave me an incorrect diagnosis. But thank you. Truly, thank you. My sister said I'd like you! I am not at all afraid to talk with you, Dr. Hall."

"You are so dear, Mrs. Azim, and yes you have been poorly treated. I'm sure your doctors didn't mean to, and God knows I have missed things too. But really, this one isn't so hard. And if you wish, please call me Prudence, like all my clients do."

Mrs. Azim's face lights up. "That is lovely, Prudence. Thank you so much, and please call me Anne—that's what my friends call me."

"It will be with pleasure, Anne, and I'm honored to be amongst your friends. Now let's treat you. I'd like to begin by putting you on a natural thyroid hormone called Nature-Throid, a combination of T4 and T3, which are both thyroid hormones. Does that sound okay to you?"

"I want to feel well again, but I have been told that once you start taking thyroid pills you can never stop. Is that right?"

I shake my head, "No. That is a common belief, but untrue. We'll begin with a very small dose, while at the same time work to heal your thyroid gland so it will function better. It you ever don't want to take the thyroid hormone, you can stop. We'll heal the thyroid gland by taking iodine, decreasing any kind of toxicity you might be exposed to, eating a special diet for thyroid health, and using immune enhancers.

"Most patients are prescribed Synthroid, Levoxyl, or Levothyroxine, which are synthetic T4 preparations. But the active thyroid hormone that causes your body to function better is T3. When only T4 is prescribed, many people never break it down to the active T3 hormone. Are you with me so far?"

"Absolutely," Anne says with a warm smile.

"Good. That's why I like to prescribe T4 plus T3. The iodine I am prescribing will help you make more of your own T4 and T3 hormones. Iodine is also a critical mineral in preventing thyroid nodules, cysts, and cancer, as well as uterine fibroids and endometriosis. Our naturopath will help you with your thyroid healing diet. I think we should do a quick thyroid ultrasound too. Do you want us to do that today, or would you rather have it done back in Dubai?"

"Please, if we can do it here, I'd be very grateful. My friend's son, who is only twenty-three, was recently diagnosed with thyroid cancer."

My eyes soften. "I am so sorry! It can happen at any age and I diagnose it several times a month. Last year, one of my young nurses decided to have our ultrasound tech check her thyroid gland and found out she had cancer. She then checked the tech's thyroid, and she also had thyroid cancer. We are seeing a real epidemic of thyroid cancer which iodine helps prevent."

Before we part, I tell Anne I won't forget her desire to reconnect to herself with new zest and passion for life. Our Center recognizes that radiant health comes from the spirit of a person, not just the physical body. We hug warmly, and I once again feel blessed by being invited to participate in the lives of my clients. It is such a privilege to help each person embark on a unique path back to her true essence.

> *"We are seeing a real epidemic of thyroid cancer, and iodine helps prevent it."*

Dr Nikki, one of our Naturopathic doctors, takes Anne into her office, and I learn later they have a lively discussion about a gluten-free diet, digestive healing, probiotics and enzymes.

> *Our Center recognizes that radiant health comes from the spirit of a person, not just the physical body.*

Anne's final consult today is with Anil Chandwani who will discuss her stress and teach her practices to help manage it. Anil is a master teacher working with our *Path of Fulfillment* program. Each time I say "Path of Fulfillment" I smile and feel happy, because it took me a very long time to name this branch of our Center.

Here's what the program is about:

"The Path of Fulfillment is the Hall Center's ongoing series of lectures, workshops and individual sessions to deepen and explore who you are. It guides you in developing fulfilling meditative and spiritual practices for vibrant health and emotional joy. This program helps you navigate life's challenging transitions in your relationships, careers, and health. Offered by a series of masters from around the world, the Path of Fulfillment inspires you to live your most expanded, conscious and fulfilling life."

> *I raised my thyroid a bit two weeks ago like you told me to, and I am really a different person.*

As Anne begins to recover and have more energy for her own life, I am relieved she will have Anil's guidance. Anil's specialty is asking clients "what's missing" in their lives and then helping them create it. Part of the physical body is our mind, which creates our thoughts and emotions. Research shows that positive and happy thoughts add seven to ten years to our life; therefore a longevity program must address this aspect of health.

My next consult with Anne is a month later. She is back in Dubai, so we're doing our session on the phone. My nurse who conducted her two-week check-in call has already told me she is doing better. Dr. Nikki has also spoken to me of her good progress.

"Hello, dear Anne! I am happy to hear your voice. How are you doing?"

"Oh, Prudence, I am so much better. I raised my thyroid a bit two weeks ago like you told me to, and I am really a different person. That small increase made such a difference. I can't believe this! I have energy, my mind is retaining all kinds of information, and I feel so much happier. Really, I feel like I am 50 percent back to myself. And that is really much, much better. I no longer feel like I am dying."

My heart feels so full. "I am so happy! That's really great news, but I want to make sure you don't feel nervous or jittery from your thyroid hormones. Some people feel shaky, or they tremble or feel their heart pounding. Have you experienced any of that?"

"Oh, is that what's been causing those symptoms? I thought it was due to drinking too much caffeine, so I cut back."

I hear a small chuckle.

"Good job with that. Lots of people start drinking more coffee because their thyroid is low, but when I correct their thyroid they realize they don't need as much coffee. But also, the T3 in Nature-Throid can cause the heart to flutter. Sometimes it can be scary and feel like you're having a heart attack. We don't want anything like that going on in this initial adjustment phase."

"No, no, it's not bad at all. I wouldn't have commented on it, except you mentioned it. I remember my patient educator telling me about it and even pointing it out in my manual … but I forgot. I guess my brain wasn't working as well as it is now." She laughs with real delight at her improved memory.

When someone has a thyroid problem that is adequately corrected, they recover at lightning speed. I love hearing from these patients! They lose excess weight, regrow their hair, stop feeling depressed, and get their energy back. The cold hands and feet, which are so common, also warm up. Correcting a thyroid deficiency can make awful symptoms just disappear. Clients come to me with what seems like multiple complex and diverse problems, but so often all of those problems stem from a thyroid problem.

I remember that when I was correcting my own thyroid levels, I was at a conference on the East Coast and it was snowing outside. For the first time in a number of years I was able to walk outside without being severely cold. Sure, I was wearing a big coat, but in the past I would always be cold, no matter what I wore. It was so wonderful to be toasty

> *When someone has a thyroid problem that is adequately corrected, they recover at lightning speed.*

and warm under the starry night. It's necessary to go slowly when rebuilding thyroid hormone back to normal levels, and there is usually an adjustment phase. Just as it took a long time for the thyroid condition to develop, it takes time to restore the hormone back to their youthful levels. Rushing this process means patients don't feel as well as when we go slowly.

I continue my conversation with Anne. "It's just wonderful you're feeling so much better. What about your dry skin and hair?"

"Well, it's a little bit better. I look less haggard and dried up, but I know that takes time, doesn't it?"

I nod my head. "Yes, the thyroid hormones have to get into your cells and start creating healthier proteins. Those healthy cells make you look and feel more beautiful. I call this beauty from the inside out. But you'll see a big difference in another few months. Promise."

"Well, even if I don't look that much better, I feel a lot better. And how I *think* I look is almost as important as how I *actually* look." We laugh together.

"Anne, I rechecked all your hormones again and discovered that your thyroid condition is called Hashimoto's. When we discover thyroid abnormalities, I always check a bit deeper to try to determine why. Have you heard about this condition?"

"No, is it cancer?" I hear the worry in her voice.

> *How I think I look is almost as important as how I actually look.*

"No, no ... no worries about cancer. It is a type of autoimmune condition that causes your body to reject your own thyroid gland. Your body's own protective antibodies attack your thyroid gland, somehow believing the thyroid gland is foreign tissue. We need to stop it right away, because you don't want your body's primary defense turned against itself. Those missiles need to be directed at cancer cells and other parasites, not your own body. The good news is that we have diagnosed the condition, and in fact have been treating it from our first consult. Gluten is a real culprit with Hashimoto's disease. It is very hard to heal the thyroid gland when anyone continues to eat gluten. How are you doing with your thyroid healing diet?"

"No problem. I was so desperate that I told Dr. Nikki I would eat exactly how she told me to, and I have. There are almost no gluten-free products in Dubai yet, but there's plenty of great food I can eat. I eat salads, meat, chicken, hummus, fruit, nuts, seeds, and a protein shake for breakfast. Really, I'm perfect."

"Anne, you are being so good. I really am proud of you. You are going to feel like you did at thirty. It just takes time to get back to 100 percent. I was wondering, do you have any mercury amalgams in your teeth?"

"No, my teeth are really good. I don't have a single filling."

I shift in my chair. "Great! The thyroid gland can be affected by mercury, but other environmental sources can cause high mercury levels as well as amalgams. I wasn't so lucky, Anne. I had to replace a number of amalgams years ago. It took months to slowly remove them all … and I had mercury under several crowns where the dentist had just capped over them. So, I'm happy you don't have to worry about your teeth. Let's do a six-hour heavy metal urine test to make sure other sources of heavy metals are not involved."

"I'm so relieved to hear that. And really I feel better already. I'm no longer scared about dementia. Prudence, I want to go out and enjoy my life again. I am still a bit tired, but if I continue to improve like I have up to this point, I'll have plenty of energy soon."

I speak with Anne again at the three-month mark, and she exudes happiness. "I can't begin to tell you how grateful I am. I feel like myself again and am filled with energy. My youngest son can't believe what has happened to me. We are actually spending quite a bit of time together. He doesn't want to go into the family business, so we are investigating what we love in life. Anil helped me to see that I had given up a lot of my life, really for nothing. I had forgotten that I went into interpreting because I loved being part of a bigger global community. My son and I have planned some summer trips because my husband and older son are so busy. We're going to India. And Bali. I listened to Deva Premal and Mitten on Mentors Channel, and I am going to one of their concerts and workshops."

Anne is referring to our chairman, Doron Libshtein, who also is the founder of Mentors Channel. He is constantly resourcing the Center with the many mentors he works with.

"That's just wonderful, Anne. I love them, too!" I smile as memories flash through my mind. "I heard them in India for the first time many years ago, and then in Santa Monica, and recently at a fabulous concert in Israel. You are in for such a treat! I wish I could go too!"

"Oh, come with us! Really, it would be wonderful."

I laugh in delight at the idea, but decline her spontaneous enthusiasm. "Anne, you are on to something with your love of travel. Keep your eyes wide open and notice what you specifically love about your trips. I would love for you to tell me you are so excited by how much people all over the world are alike, that you have started a One People Foundation—or something amazing like that. Or that you are fascinated by plant medicine and have enrolled in an Ayurveda healing program to become an Ayurvedic doctor. Really, your heart will lead you. And Anil will guide you if you get stuck."

Anne laughs in delight. "Okay, I'll do both of those things. They would both interest me. Prudence, I am just so happy to be back in the world."

⌾

I have a session with Anne's sister a few months later. She is doing so well that we make only a few adjustments, but what she really wants to talk about is having her sister back again! They have been traveling together— hiking up to remote monasteries in Thailand and taking cooking classes at Kamalaya—a luscious wellness resort owned by my dear friends. Anne's energy sounds fantastic. She

> *"It was really just my thyroid, because everything is back to normal; my skin is great, and my hair is growing again. I have energy and a new drive."*

definitely doesn't sound like the same woman I began treating only five months ago.

⌾

At our six-month meeting, I talk with Anne in person. Bubbling with energy, she confirms what her sister told me.

"You were right, Prudence." Her smile lights up the room. "It was really just my thyroid, because everything is back to normal. My skin is great and my hair is growing again. I have energy and a new drive. I am never depressed and, even though you told me to slowly wean off my Celexa, I knew I had to get off it right away. So I just stopped … how do you Americans say? Cold turkey. Is that right? Yes, just cold turkey. I have been off it for three months, since right after our last talk."

"And you're okay? No anxiety or anything?"

Anne nods. "It wasn't the right treatment for what caused the depression, so I knew I'd be better off without it. It stopped my sex drive and kept me down. My husband is still not spending that much time with me because he's so busy, but he keeps up with what I'm doing. And he's being much nicer. Or maybe I am being nicer to him, which makes him sweeter to me. But I do feel sexier and am again making love with him once in a while. I don't know what will happen with us, but he's a good man. And if I'm true to myself, keeping up my own interests, there's a good chance he might join me traveling sometime. I am writing a book about my travels, because the more I notice what I like, the more I want to share my observations. I am titling it, *The Call of Distant Lands: A Muslim Woman's Return to Herself.* It's about the people I meet, actually a reflection of who I am, a mirror of my heart. I'm surprised that other women seem quite interested in it. Maybe I am meant to be some kind of guide for women. I liked the movie 'Eat, Pray,

> *It is fairly common for women to become hypothyroid after the birth of a child, due to the mother's iodine being depleted by the fetus's needs.*

Love.' My journey feels a bit like that." I smile, knowing her journey has taken off in full flight.

I think back to my own thyroid problems. After the birth of my first baby, I had two miscarriages in quick succession. I immediately thought the miscarriages could be due to a hypothyroid condition.

It is fairly common for women to become hypothyroid after the birth of a child, due to the mother's iodine being depleted by the fetus's needs. But my blood work was consistently normal, except for low estrogen levels due to the fact that I was still nursing my baby. But I had too many symptoms of being hypothyroid to consider myself normal. I was tired, losing my hair, having difficulty maintaining my weight, and feeling kind of blue. On top of those symptoms, I was freezing! My body just didn't stay warm. Even though this was right at the beginning of my gynecology career, I knew I didn't want to miscarry again due to such a correctable cause. I decided to take a small amount of thyroid and see how I felt. When I did, I felt a light bulb turn back on in my body. I warmed up, felt new energy and happiness, and went on to have two more children. Just like my patients tell me, "It is a miracle!"

I had too many symptoms of being hypothyroid to consider myself normal. I was tired, losing my hair, having difficulty maintaining my weight, and feeling kind of blue.

I also starting taking iodine and eliminated gluten from my diet, and I haven't experienced any further problems. I take three grains of Nature-thyroid based on the results of my twenty-four hour urine tests and Thyroflex scores. My blood levels are elevated above the "normal" ranges, but my numbers are similar to other clients whose thyroid is clinically balanced. I feel good with no symptoms of hypothyroidism, no bone loss, and no heart palpitations.

A client with the aforementioned maladies may not have the complex conditions she has been diagnosed with—like chronic fatigue or fibromyalgia. She might, instead, have the disease of chronic misdiagnosis.

Thyroid is such a simple diagnosis to make if you know what you are looking for. Many patients already suspect they have thyroid deficiency, but can't find a doctor to confirm it. Some of these patients have other problems, such as adrenal deficiency or menopause. But more frequently than not, they are absolutely correct. Due to the Internet, it is wonderful how educated patients are these days. A simple prescription for low thyroid can change a patient's life, and the prescription is inexpensive and available in every pharmacy.

A client with the above mentioned maladies may not have the complex conditions she has been diagnosed with—like chronic fatigue or fibromyalgia. She might, instead, have the disease of chronic misdiagnosis. Misdiagnosis is exactly what has happened to hundreds of patients who have ended up in my office, their thyroid condition having been missed for many long and painful years.

Thyroid is such a simple diagnosis to make if you know what you are looking for.

Takeaway:

The diagnosis of thyroid disease is missed in 50 to 60 percent of cases when a physician relies only on a blood test. While blood testing needs to be done, other tests are more accurate. (Blood testing includes TSH, free T3, free T4, reverse T3, and thyroid antibodies.) The FDA-approved Thyroflex reflex test is quick and 95 percent accurate in diagnosing thyroid conditions. Twenty-four hour urine testing is also a very accurate diagnostic tool for this condition.

Symptoms of low thyroid:

Symptoms help to correctly diagnose thyroid conditions. The most common symptoms are: fatigue; weight gain; poor memory; depression; hair loss; poor nail quality; dry, cracking skin; puffy hands, feet and eyes; constipation; heavier menses; and loss of the outer edges of the eyebrow. To help you diagnose whether or not you have thyroid disease, I have included a quiz for you to take.

Please score the following symptoms using the 4 possible responses

0 = never / I do not experience that / I don't know the answer

1 = mild / occasionally / a little bit

2 = moderate / frequently / quite a bit

3 = severe / constantly / a lot!

- Do you have cold hands and feet?
- Are you tired when waking up in the morning?
- Are you tired throughout the day?
- Are you gaining weight or having trouble losing it?
- Are you depressed or feel sad?
- Do you have decreased vitality?
- Is your brain foggy?
- Is your skin or hair dry?
- Are you losing hair?
- Are the outer edges of your eyebrows thin?
- Are your hands, feet or eyelids puffy?
- Are you constipated?
- Do you get muscle spasms / cramps?

If you score ten or more symptoms on the quiz, there is an excellent chance your thyroid hormones are deficient.

My prescription for your thyroid:

- Nature-Throid, Westroid and Armour are all natural combinations of thyroid hormones containing both T3 and T4. They require a prescription. Begin with a quarter to a half-grain and titrate up slowly until you reach a normal Thyroflex score and general sense of well-being.
- 1 Biodine capsule daily for iodine supplementation. This is not a prescription and helps the thyroid gland function more effectively.

- 4-5 Brazil nuts a day contain selenium, which helps the thyroid gland function better.

- Gluten-free diet and anti-inflammatory foods

- Repeat Thyroflex reflex test, questionnaire, and lab work six to eight weeks after the initial test to adjust doses.

Chapter 5

Weight Loss

It is wintertime in Los Angeles and we are experiencing a rare period of cold weather. The wind howls outside, bringing bitter cold to everything it touches. I am reminded of living in Majorca, Spain, when I was in high school. The winters were so cold, with icy winds whipping off the Mediterranean Sea. My parents bought all five of us children warm sheepskin jackets, but they didn't keep the cold away. At lunchtime, We would hurry to the nearby Spanish Bodega cafe and huddle around the fireplace to drink hot chocolate.

> *"I just can't stop gaining weight. I eat 1200 calories a day, exercise 5 days a week and still, I can't lose a pound."*

During this winter revelry, Melanie comes to the Center for her first consult, bundled up and red cheeked, but with a forlorn expression splattered on her face. After introductions and my invitation to talk, she jumps right in.

"I just can't stop gaining weight. I eat 1200 calories a day, exercise 5 days a week and still, I can't lose a pound. I feel so frustrated I could just cry. In fact I do cry, and I hate myself for being like this. How could this happen to me?" Her voice rises to a sad crescendo, then drops to a whimper.

Poor Melanie! She is so pretty, but when she unbundles her big coat, I see how uncomfortable she is in her body, cramped into tight clothes with noticeable bulges. Her hair appears dry and thin. She carries the bulk of the weight in her mid-abdominal area. She actually carries the weight quite well, but, judging by her appearance, she is about fifty pounds overweight.

I reach out my hand in support. "I am so sorry you are suffering like this, Melanie. You don't deserve it, not even a little bit. How did it all start?"

"I have always battled a bit with my weight." She slumps against the back of her chair. "I'd gain and lose the same ten pounds over and over again. I gained twenty pounds during my first year in college—the freshman bulge, they called it. I lost most of it the second year. In my late twenties I broke my leg and gained a sizeable amount of weight. I was never able to take off those twenty-five pounds, but I was still active and looked good. I got married at thirty, and then I really gained weight during my pregnancies—fifty pounds with the first baby and about

> *"So many doctors concentrate on the calories a person eats and how much exercise they do. This is not the only way to approach weight loss. We need to go deeper than that."*

seventy-five with the second baby. The scale just won't budge. I have done Jenny Craig, Weight Watchers, diet pills and even the HCG diet last year. It was wonderful! I lost forty pounds, but it all came back, plus another five. Now I am fifty-five pounds overweight. My kids are now ten and twelve years old. Isn't it time to finally have my thin body back?"

I completely understand. "You have really been in a big battle for many years, haven't you? And it must feel horrible to be starving yourself with no results."

"Yes, it's like a battle, and I'm so sick of it. I really just hate myself. I am constantly in a dialogue with myself: 'Don't eat that. Stop being so bad. You'll be sorry. How can you be so weak?' Prudence, I really punish myself, and the worst thing is that every time I eat the tiniest 'bad' food, I gain weight. And I'm not eating foods that are really all that bad, and I don't overeat very often."

"What do you consider bad food?" I ask.

"Well, it could be a piece of bread with turkey on it, or maybe a bowl of cereal, and when I do eat those foods I make sure I exercise a bit harder than usual. I do a P90X routine, which is pretty intense, but I can still gain a few pounds. This is crazy!"

I hear this kind of story several times a week, so I jump right in to try and educate Melanie as to what's really going on with her body. "So many doctors concentrate on the calories a person eats and how much exercise they do. This is not the only way to approach weight loss. We need to go deeper than that. Did you ever take the birth control pill?"

"Yes, I did as a freshman in college, but I stopped over the summer because I thought maybe it had something to do with my weight gain. When I married, I took it again for five years. Do you think the weight gain had something to do with the pill?"

"Hormones are critical in maintaining the body's ideal composition, and yes, the pill upsets the pituitary gland's balance and can set women up for weight gain. We have so much to talk about, Melanie. Not being able to lose weight has nine major causes. It's like a pie with nine pieces and each piece causes weight gain."

"Well, I'm glad there are causes for this because, frankly, I feel like giving up. How many pie pieces do I have?" She looks at me with hopeful eyes.

> *The pill upsets the pituitary gland's balance and can set women up for weight gain.*

"Well, you actually only have four pieces . . . but you could have had all nine, so I'm happy we won't have to work quite so hard. Let's begin by looking at your blood tests. One of the tests measured your sugar and insulin, which comes from your pancreas. Melanie, your test indicates you are almost diabetic. It's next to impossible to lose weight when you are pre-diabetic. Has anyone told you this before?"

> *"Not being able to lose weight has nine major causes. It's like a pie with nine pieces, and each piece causes weight gain."*

"NO! Melanie shakes her head in disbelief. "Almost diabetic, and I just had my blood drawn six months ago … again. I am so upset about my weight gain. I can't believe no one told me anything about this problem. I have actually seen three other doctors over the past five years trying to find help."

I reach out and touch her arm. "I am so sorry, honey. I really am. When I trained at USC, I wasn't actually taught anything about weight loss. Can you believe that? I was just like all those doctors you saw. In my first few months in private practice, about half my patients asked me how to lose weight. I really had no idea what to do, because they didn't seem to be eating a lot of calories, so I had to literally figure this out. In fact, I studied it extensively, and the answers didn't come from only one medical specialty—they came from many. I have now helped thousands of patients achieve their ideal weight. In your situation, this pre-diabetic condition means your metabolism has been damaged from high blood sugar. When you eat carbohydrates or sugar, insulin pours out of the pancreas, picks up the sugar and brings it into the cells for energy. However, in your case, the cells already have too much sugar, which causes the cells to become resistant to insulin. It's like the government wanting to put nuclear waste storage in rural areas, and those little towns rebel and refuse to be dumped on. It's the same with toxic sugar—the cells refuse to accept it."

> *"It's next to impossible to lose weight when you are pre-diabetic."*

"What happens to the sugar when the cells won't take it?" Melanie asks with genuine interest.

> *You have both high cholesterol and high blood sugar. Both conditions make weight loss difficult.*

"Good question, and the answer is one of the reasons you've gained weight. When the cells are too saturated with sugar, it has to be dumped somewhere else. The brain receives a huge amount of it because it doesn't have a barrier to keep it out like other cells do. The rest is put into the liver. The liver stores as much as it can, and turns the rest into cholesterol. These triglycerides and cholesterol are then released back into the bloodstream which raises cholesterol levels. The body is smart and knows that too much sugar is more dangerous than too much cholesterol. Melanie, you have both high cholesterol and high blood sugar. Both conditions make weight loss difficult. Imagine that in one arm you have an IV pumping sugar into you 24/7, and in the other an IV infusing fat. That is certainly not a good scenario for weight loss. We have to turn this situation around, so I'm going to give you a supplement I formulated called Sugar Balance. Our nutritionist is also going to help you with this."

Melanie looks hopeful and asks what her other three pieces of pie are. "I wish I could eat those pieces of pie!"

I laugh. "Well, they are eating you! Pie piece number two is food allergies. See your gluten test? Sky high! When you eat foods you're allergic to like bread and cereal, it sets up an inflammatory reaction in your body—and inflammation causes weight gain. It also causes all kinds of dreaded diseases. Weight gain is not caused only by the number of calories you eat; even more important is the quality of the calories."

"I have only been counting calories. I thought a calorie was a calorie. But I know all about gluten," Melanie exclaims. "My sister eats a gluten-free diet. I can't believe I need to be doing the same thing."

> *Weight gain is not caused only by the number of calories you eat; even more important is the quality of the calories.*

"Well, you probably share one of her same genes. It's a genetic problem that family members have. In fact, whole nations can be gluten intolerant. For example, the Irish tend to carry the genes."

"My grandfather is Irish … well, English." Melanie muses.

"The English frequently carry the gene too, but we are all so mixed up in terms of heritage that anyone can carry gluten genes. I have two of them."

"So you can't eat gluten?"

"That's right. I have been gluten-free for twenty years. It was initially hard to give up because I love Italian food and used to eat pasta and bread, but I had to stop. When my mother died of Alzheimer's disease, I realized I had been far too lenient with myself about inflammation, which is one of its causes. I eliminated gluten, because I knew I was intolerant to it. I stopped cold, and you can too. We'll walk with you—and you won't be alone."

> *You definitely have undiagnosed low thyroid, which is a major cause of your weight gain.*

Melanie's smile lights up the room. "Wow, I can't believe all this. You're like a detective. I'll do it. I really will come off gluten. What are the other pie pieces?"

I glance at her chart. "Well, your thyroid is low. Your symptoms are subtle. Your blood work is normal, but I can see it in your Thyroflex test. And you indicated thirty-two low thyroid symptoms on your questionnaire, which is critical. Most doctors don't seriously take into account how a patient feels. You definitely have undiagnosed low thyroid, which is a major cause of your weight gain. We need to give you a small amount of natural thyroid hormone and some iodine to help your thyroid gland be healthier."

Melanie nods her head and agrees to take both after I explain that it is a natural treatment that we will try and heal her gland with, and she might not have to take them forever.

"Our last piece of the weight gain pie is that you have an intestinal parasite, which is why you're so bloated, along with the gluten allergy, which causes weight gain. Any time you have parasites or bugs in the digestive tract it causes inflammation, autoimmune diseases and more. We'll have to do some gut healing with you. You'll need some herbs to kill the parasite and some probiotics and enzymes. Actually, there's quite a lot to unravel. But can you see why weight loss isn't just calories in/calories out?"

"Oh, my God, I can't believe all the doctors and nutritionists I've seen who just limited my calories and made me exercise. I'll sometimes exercise two hours a day and literally eat nothing. Yes, I see why that hasn't been working, but I've been blaming myself for so many years—really hating myself."

> *"Any time you have parasites or bugs in the digestive tract it causes inflammation, autoimmune diseases and more."*

"I am so sorry." I feel so much empathy for her. I see patients every day who have felt the same. "Really, this isn't your fault. It happened to me too. After I had my first baby I couldn't lose my pregnancy weight. Even though it wasn't the end of the world I felt miserable. I normally weigh 128 pounds, but I kept hovering at my pregnancy weight of 148. I had to take myself on as a patient. I found out my thyroid was low and, just like you, my sugar was quite high. I was a vegetarian and ate a lot of gluten-free pasta and rice—comfort food, because I was so stressed. It just wasn't good for me so I had to completely change my style of eating. But back to you, dear Melanie. Your weight gain is due to high blood sugar (insulin resistance), gluten intolerance, an intestinal parasite and low thyroid. And although there are several causes, they are all treatable."

Melanie's eyes moisten. "Prudence, I feel real hope."

"We're going to resolve this for sure! There's always a big emotional component to eating that we'll address. We have feelings, preferences, and blocks to our success. But let's take you to our Naturopath, Dr. Petra, who is our weight loss specialist. She'll help set up this gut-healing, sugar-busting, gluten-free program I've prescribed, and I'll give you some natural thyroid, iodine and Sugar Balance. We're going to lick this thing. Promise."

A month later Melanie returns, beaming with happiness. "I have so much more energy! I actually *feel* like exercising. I was doing it before, but really I was dragging myself around."

"That is fantastic! How is being gluten free?"

"Well, it's hard. I cheated a few times but felt so bad I'm not going to eat gluten again. But the good news is I lost eight pounds! I'm not constipated and the bloating has gone down."

"This weight loss should be permanent, unlike other diet plans. Look at how much your sugar has fallen!"

Melanie's eyes light up. "I still have further to go, but it's a lot better."

"Yes! We've now cracked your weight loss code, so let's help you stay on track. Your Thyroflex score is better, but still not in the ideal range. You need a bit more thyroid. Are you having any bad symptoms from it, like nervousness or heart flutters?"

"Nope, nothing bad is happening. I feel good, and I'm taking the iodine at night."

"Great. Let's double the thyroid pills, which will really help. Have you been working with your weight loss coach?"

"Absolutely!" Melanie sits up straight in her chair. "I have an appointment every week, email my food journal twice a week, and when I freak out because I've eaten desert or something, I email her for help. She's taught me all about emotional eating and relaxing in the middle of cravings. But I don't have many cravings now with Sugar Balance. One thing that has helped a lot is that I had three meetings with Priya, your mind-body teacher. I love her! She helped me see how I was constantly being a dictator with each bite I took. I was being so mean to myself. I am now much more aware of it and can stop it quickly. That's helped me in a big way to control my binge eating."

"Excellent, Priya is very wise and insightful. I love her too. Are you getting some massages? It really helps break up the fat and release toxins. And you're drinking large amounts of water, right?"

"Yep, ten glasses between meals, but I haven't had time for a massage. I will though—as my reward. I feel like I'm really making progress with my goals!"

Melanie continues to work with her coach each week. They are dealing with all kinds of issues and have cut dairy out of her diet, as well as eggs, because she seems intolerant to them. She's drinking a shake for breakfast and has two totally green days a week, including a green shake. She is using our fabulous digestive enzymes (LiyfZymes) to heal her digestion issues.

Melanie returns for an appointment at three months. Wow! She looks so little. I hadn't realized she is so diminutive. The weight has fallen off her, and she offers me a shy smile.

"Hi, little Melanie, is this what you've been hiding? You look about six years old."

"Well, I do feel kind of vulnerable without all my weight. I've lost thirty-two pounds. Can you believe it? I was beginning to sabotage myself, but last month I resumed my sessions with Priya. Really, I'm having some good talks with her about who's in charge of me—my mind or my heart? I feel much less anxious and I'm growing in respect for myself. I also love meditating with Anil each week at the Center and now have a supportive group of friends. My kids like to come with me once in a while too, which is really great. I'm now more of a leader for them. But I don't know about my husband—he kind of hasn't noticed me yet."

"Oh, I didn't know you were having problems. What's going on?"

"Well, he's been so grumpy and angry the last two months. I thought it was because I was being the food police with everyone, but I think it's more than that. He's just angry with me. I don't get it. I am so much better in all ways."

"Do you think he is threatened by how beautiful you are becoming? Men sometimes feel an attractive wife will be taken away from them. Is he approaching you sexually?"

"Almost never; he just keeps saying he's too tired."

"Well, maybe he has hormone problems too. Would he come in?" Melanie isn't sure, but said she'd have a conversation with him. She really loves him.

I'm delighted to see Thomas come in two weeks later with Melanie. He is indeed exhausted and grumpy. He is also about 80 pounds overweight. He tells me he used to weigh 190, and now he is pushing 270. He was an athlete in college, but with all the pressure he's under, he has no time to exercise. His labs show he has low testosterone levels and terribly deficient adrenal hormones due to stress. He's the owner of a pipe and air duct firm, which turns out to be a complex and demanding business with lots of hours and travel back and forth to China.

I prescribe Mega Adrenal, which is a bioidentical hormone and herb supplement to help his adrenal glands return to normal, instruct him on how to give himself testosterone injections each week, and also help him sleep with Sweet Sleep and Melatonin. He agrees to see the naturopath, which will take Melanie out of the role of being his instructor. (Men usually hate that.) His blood sugar is also high, so we will tailor a nutrition program for his unique needs. For men, raising testosterone levels, managing stress, eating healthy foods and good workouts overwhelmingly cause major weight loss. Men come back in three or four months looking ripped—like youngsters. And why not? Our body likes to be healthy and strong.

I receive a surprise video from Melanie and Thomas six months later on their wedding anniversary. Melanie looks amazing and recites a poem she wrote for the occasion about her way back home to herself and her childhood sweetheart. She is so dreamy in her summer dress, really radiant. Then Thomas speaks about how she is still the same sweetheart she always was, and that he's now able to meet her. He speaks in such a loving way and actually looks like a different man from the one I initially met, as he's a good fifty pounds lighter. They cut the cake and the film ends. Melanie has included a little note:

Dear Prudence,

Can you believe I've lost fifty-three pounds? That's enough for now, because I feel just right. I don't have the old feeling of not being thin enough. It is really incredible how happy we both are, with Thomas back to his old self and championing me in my health and not fighting me like he used to do. I am traveling some with him while the kids are in camp, and I have so much more energy.

My diet is no problem. I can't eat gluten at all, (that was a gluten-free cake in the video) but I eat some eggs once in a while. Dairy just doesn't agree with me, so I don't miss it. I know you are aware of most of this, but you might not know I am learning to be a meditation teacher. I've been through so much myself that I really want to help others. I didn't know that I am a natural teacher. I've had some good teachers around me!

Thank you from the bottom of my heart. I have found my way back from such a place of loneliness, and all along this path, I never felt alone. Please use my story in any way you can to help others. I am just so grateful, I feel like crying. I have an appointment in six months so I'll see you soon.

Yours,

Melanie

When Melanie came to see me six months later she had lost another ten pounds, but she didn't seem to want to talk much about her weight. She did want to make sure her cholesterol was good (it was perfect) and her sugar down (also perfect). She was way too busy to make weight and food the focus in her life. She was so impressed by the work Priya had done with her that she started studying with her to become a teacher herself, and was already building herself a little practice. Good girl, Melanie. Way to be an example!

My next weight loss patient comes to me with very different circumstances. Brenda, an attorney, fifty-seven, is of African American descent, and is overweight. She begins to pour out her heart.

"I have my own law practice and am handling big cases. I don't know what it feels like *not* to be stressed. I can't seem to sleep. My mind won't stop. But Prudence, the worst thing is that my weight keeps going up. I can't keep doing this. I look like my mother, and I'm not feeling very sexy either." She looks at me expectantly.

"Well, Counselor," I tease her, "tell that to the judge. You look very sexy, and even though you are a bit overweight, you are beautiful. You could be a model."

Brenda laughs and her eyes crinkle in the most charming way. "Okay, okay, tell me what to do. I am forty-five pounds overweight and am ready to be a sexy model. The stress from all this attorney stuff is getting kind of old. I need a little … or maybe a big … change in my life."

"I understand the need for a change in life, bringing in new energies and new ideas. And yes, I agree that all your stress is really affecting you. Look at how low your stress hormones are. You are pretty burned out." I open Brenda's new patient binder to the section on stress. Her four hormones are all way below the normal range.

> *"Doctors talk about women being 'post-menopausal,' but the truth of the matter is that if you don't replace your hormones to youthful levels, you are in menopause for the rest of your life."*

"I knew it! Prudence, I am just so tired. When I have a bit of extra stress, like when I'm in court for a few days, I have to force myself to get out of bed."

Brenda rates her fatigue as a three on a scale of one to ten, with ten having the most energy. A three is really low, but consistent with all four of her stress hormones being so low.

I glance up at her. "Brenda, when did you go into menopause? Your estradiol is so low, and so is your testosterone. Both are due to menopause."

"My menopause was pretty bad eight or nine years ago, but I'm through it now. The hot flashes are all gone."

"Oh, Brenda, I would love you to be through menopause, but that's not the way it works. Doctors talk about women being 'post-menopausal,' but the truth of the matter is that if you don't replace your hormones to youthful levels, you are in menopause for the rest of your life. Did you know that women in their forties and early fifties gain about thirty to forty pounds due to perimenopause and menopause?" Her eyes tell me she fully understands what I'm saying.

"In your case, the causes of your weight gain are stress, including your work and not sleeping, your menopause, and I also think you may be depleted due to too much exercise. What is your exercise routine?"

"Well, most days I'm up at 4:30 to exercise. I run, then do the P90X, but I wouldn't say it's too much. Obviously, isn't enough because I keep gaining weight."

"I think it might be just the opposite! If you're already stressed, which causes weight gain, and then you add more stress by exercising vigorously, it worsens the stress imbalance and causes more weight gain. While your adrenals heal, I would like you to try restorative exercise, like yoga."

"Sure, but I pulled a hamstring, so I am strengthening it by running."

"You can probably go back to a bit of running when you're more healed. But to resolve this weight problem, we need to think differently than most doctors. We need to address root causes. First and most importantly, we need to take you out of menopause with bioidentical hormones. Do you know anything about them?"

> *"If you're already stressed, which causes weight gain, and then you add more stress by exercising vigorously, it worsens the stress imbalance and causes more weight gain."*

"Absolutely. I have read all of Suzanne Somers' books, and that's one reason I'm here."

"Great!" I smile warmly. "I am so happy to hear that. Let's give you a little estrogen and testosterone cream to begin with, and also my Super Adrenal mixture. Super Adrenal is a real miracle combination to replace your adrenal hormones and help heal your glands. Sleeplessness also stresses your adrenal glands, causing more weight gain, so let's give you a few natural sleep remedies. We can help you identify your stress by wearing a WellBe watch, like the one I'm wearing. I wear mine all the time because it gives me a signal when my stress is elevated, making me aware of what's happening. Then it gives me a solution to immediately lower the stress. I refer to my watch as a "him" because it feels like WellBe is protecting me from an evil dragon, or something like that. He's cute isn't he?"

> *The WellBe not only identifies when you're stressed, it also gives you a quick solution to immediately end it. Thank you Mentors Channel for creating it!*

Brenda asks if she can wear it and after it's adjusted to her the initial reading tells us she is 88 percent stressed. The solution WellBe chooses for her is thirty seconds of quiet breathing. Her stress plummets to 27 percent—much better!

"Wow, I am totally game." Brenda claps her hands with delight. "I'm just surprised no one told me how stress was causing me to gain weight. I've been having food delivered because my doctor said I'd lose weight that way, but I haven't … not at all."

"I understand. I think differently about weight loss." I touch her hand. "Yes, food is important, but it's not only about the calories, it's also the quality of the food you eat. We need to decrease all sources of inflammation in your body, which can come from eating foods that might agitate any allergic reaction. That sets up inflammation, and so does having low estrogen in menopause. You also said your joints are hurting. We'll do an elimination diet and see what foods might be exacerbating that inflammation. Of course our natural estrogen cream is anti-inflammatory."

Brenda next sees our Naturopathic doctor who feels her digestion could be the source of her inflammation. She gives her a stool analysis kit to do at home, designs her anti-inflammatory diet, and suggests she begin some IV nutrient therapy and weekly far-infrared saunas. I touch base with her as she leaves, and she seems quite cheered.

Brenda returns in five weeks, and seems happier. She tells me she's lost five pounds. Her hormones and special diet are doing the trick, and the fatigue is also lifting due to her estrogen and adrenal healing.

"I feel better, Prudence! Maybe 20 or 30 percent better. I actually didn't realize I was feeling so bad. The extra sleep helps, but it's the hormones that are helping the most."

She now rates herself a six out of ten in terms of her energy, and she scores better on most questionnaire items. She's been doing yogi Mark Whitwell's seven-minute yoga routine each morning and using the extra morning time to sleep. This is exactly what her body needs—rest and restoration.

"Prudence, I was embarrassed to tell you before, but I used estrogen pills five years ago because my hot flashes were so bad, but I didn't lose weight like I have with your cream. I gained weight! I don't know why I had the confidence to go on them again, but I did, and it's really starting to work. I haven't lost five pounds in over eight years. I felt my body had betrayed me, but it's getting better."

"Gosh, Brenda, I am so sorry about you gaining weight on hormones before. Most of the non-bioidentical (synthetic) hormones cause enormous weight gain and have given hormones in general a bad name. Do you remember if you were on Premarin?"

Brenda nods her head. "Uh-huh. I sure was. It got rid of the hot flashes but I was still so depressed my doctor put me on Zoloft."

I scrunch up my nose. "Oh, I abhor it when doctors treat depression caused by menopause with antidepressants. It's just bad medicine, like treating a hungry child with an appetite suppressant. A menopausal body is depressed because the brain is starving for estrogen, not for Zoloft. When did you come off? Did your depression get better?"

"Oh, I forgot to write that on my intake form. I was in a rush … no, I'm still on it."

> I scrunch up my nose. "Oh, I abhor it when doctors treat depression caused by menopause with antidepressants. It's just bad medicine, like treating a hungry child with an appetite suppressant."

"This is great news, Brenda." I smile to reassure her. "If we can take you off, it's a ticket for even more weight loss. Did you know that antidepressants frequently cause weight gain?"

"I had no idea!" Her eyes grow wide. "And at this point, the most depressing thing for me is my weight. So being on it makes no sense at all. It's kind of crazy to be on an antidepressant that increases my weight, when the weight is the cause of my depression!"

I explain our depression protocol to Brenda and she agrees to give it a try. I raise her estrogen a bit because her current lab values are still quite low, and we add iodine to support her thyroid.

One month later Brenda returns, beaming. "Prudence, look at me. I'm doing it, and I feel so much better. I'm eating the way I should—not a 100 percent, but much better. I've lost ten pounds, and men are looking at me a bit more." She giggles in a sexy way.

"I am so proud of you! You truly are a beauty. There is no way men will be able to ignore you!"

Her energy level is now at a seven to eight out of ten, and she tells me she has taken Doron Libshtein's "Walk your Path" workshop on Life Fulfillment. She doesn't know where it will take her, but she is truly inspired.

My heart warms and I understand what she's experiencing. Big things happen when Doron enters someone's life. I know, because he is my mentor. Under his guidance, new books are flying out of me and the lectures are flowing; he's keeping me on track and on task with the goals I identified. I need a big life, and with Doron's help, I know where I want to go and how to get there. I smile as I consider what could happen to this dynamo named Brenda.

I add progesterone to Brenda's hormonal regimen to mimic her cycle around age thirty, add a bit more estrogen, and change the locations of her estrogen placement. Dorfsman, one of our great naturopaths, comes in to discuss Brenda's GI tract. We all decide she needs to do a detox complete with nutritional IVs, and continue with the far infrared saunas. Brenda leaves with Dorfsman to go over the plan in more detail.

In six months, I see Brenda's name on my schedule and can't wait to see her. She has been surprisingly quiet, and even though I have been getting sneak previews from the team, I haven't had a chance to catch up with her.

As I follow her back to my office, there's a defined sway of her back and her long, sexy legs … more bravely exposed, and she's so sure of herself!

"Brenda, look at you! You have become a model, just as I predicted!"

Brenda tosses back her shoulder-length hair, pulled back from her face with a fetching bandana, and laughs. "No, I haven't! I've become a politician!"

"What? And gave up your career as a super model? Well, I'm not surprised! Tell me all about it."

Brenda has been privately mentored by Doron since the conference she took with him and has identified that her life's mission is to help protect the environment. Little by little she has cut back her law practice hours and is now working 50 percent less. She has more room to breathe and has begun a second business with a lively environmental group. The group is planning a trip to the Antarctic to investigate the environmental changes causing glacier melting. She has agreed to head up a group to advise the government on environmental policy. I am so impressed! She explains that politics has been a lifelong interest of hers, and that in law school she wanted to go into an environmental field but was afraid she wouldn't be able to support herself. With Doron as her mentor, she sees her life more clearly and is back on track with what she needs to accomplish for her soul-health.

"And, Prudence, I've lost forty pounds—did you notice? It just fell off me."

"Brenda, I am so happy for you. Truly overjoyed! You look wonderful, and you obviously feel so excited about your life. Your labs are almost perfect. We can tweak things a bit, but look at your result: You're no longer in menopause and your adrenals are just great."

Brenda throws her head back and laughs. "I feel like I did at thirty, really, and I'm dating a wonderful man in my environmental group. He's so talented! He's a big environmentalist, but comes from the business side of the environmental world. He's a world traveler for his businesses, and we're trying to figure out how I'm going to travel with him without going broke. But Doron has tons of ideas to help with that!" She is beaming—and so am I.

Takeaway:

Weight loss resistance is due to the following nine major causes:

1. Imbalanced ovarian hormones due to the pill, menopause or perimenopause

2. Low thyroid conditions

3. High blood sugar: insulin resistance and diabetes

4. Life stress due to sleeplessness, over-exercising, extreme caloric restriction, work, surgeries, physical illness, and emotional factors. Wear a WellBe bracelet to identify and decrease stress. (I wear mine everyday.)

5. Digestive problems due to parasites, yeast and leaky gut

6. Food intolerances or allergies including gluten, soy, corn, dairy, sugar, eggs and many grains

7. Lifestyle factors such as overeating and lack of proper exercise

8. Toxic exposure to heavy metals

9. Medications for depression, birth control, blood pressure, hormones (if synthetic or non-bioidentical), inflammation (like prednisone), allergies and diabetes

What is the best diet? An organic, anti-inflammatory diet without grains, sugar, or dairy works best. Plenty of greens, lots of fruit, good amounts of raw food, nuts and seeds, beans, super foods, healthy oils and grass-fed protein sources are the key.

My prescription for weight loss:

- Identify the core causes of your weight loss resistance and correct each problem.

- Create a team around you to help support and inspire you.

- Wear a WellBe bracelet to monitor and decrease stress. Body Software Lepta Trim: 2 capsules per day

- Body Software Bliss: 1-2 capsules per day to help stay positive and reduce emotional eating

- Organic plant protein smoothies

- Iodine to help the thyroid function better: 10-12 mg per day

Chapter 6

Depression and Anxiety

So many of my clients are depressed and anxious, and I feel so badly for each one of them.

> *When our body chemistry is imbalanced, depression and anxiety are common.*

It's not uncommon for tears to be shed during our conversations. Clients are depressed because they don't like their bodies, can't find love, have financial or marriage problems, hate their jobs, or are facing crises with their children or aging parents. Many times they are depressed for no discernible reason. In truth, life can be pretty hard on this planet called Earth. As a hormone specialist I know that when body chemistry is imbalanced depression and anxiety are common. I also know it is not only hormone imbalances that cause depression; they can stem from poor diet, toxicity, poor digestive health, lifestyle and our soul's need to journey home to its core self.

When I first greet Deborah, I see suffering in her eyes. They are veiled in sadness, her shoulders are slumped forward and her head is bent.

I greet her warmly. "I'm so happy you have come to see me today. Get comfortable on the couch, and let's have a cup of tea. I would love to hear what's going on and how I can help."

Deborah shuffles over to the couch and plops down. After letting out a deep breath she says, "Dr. Prudence, I am in the middle of a crisis. I have heard about you for a long time but I just haven't felt well enough to actually come. But I had to this time. Really, I feel you're my last chance. Every day I feel so depressed. I cry, can't leave the house and end up watching TV all day in my room. When I decide I have to get out, I feel so anxious that I'm just immobilized. And I am so overweight! Look at me! And my sex drive is zero. I really don't even know who I am anymore."

I reach out and touch her hand. "It sounds pretty bad, Deborah, and I am so grateful you came. There is nothing more important than your being here, and I will use all the resources I have available to help you. Tell me, when did this awful depression begin?"

"It's been going on for a long time. I started getting depressed right after the birth of my second child fifteen years ago. My doctor said I had postpartum depression and started me on antidepressants right away. They helped a little bit, but not enough, because I still felt pretty down. I couldn't lose the baby weight, and that made me depressed too. Then my mother died three years ago, and I just haven't been able to recover. Every day I think about her; she was my best friend. I guess I'm next in line. I don't think I'll ever get over that loss."

"Deborah, I am so sorry about your mother and how sad you're feeling. How did your mother die?"

"She died of a sudden and unexpected heart attack. She was only sixty-seven, and I can't believe I wasn't able to say goodbye. My father is still alive and seems to have gone on with his life. He has a new girlfriend and travels a lot. I don't hold anything against him, but it doesn't seem right that he seems to have recovered when I haven't."

I smile in empathy. "Every person grieves in their own way. There's no right way or no correct timing. Has your mother come back to visit you? Has she given you any messages?"

"Well, that's an interesting question for a doctor to ask. Are you a psychic?"

"No," I say laughing, "but when I sit with patients certain things come up and I usually go with what I feel. We all have our intuitive side."

"Well, she actually has come to me several times in my dreams, and she's always cleaning the house with a broom. She keeps telling me to clean my house. 'Clean your house, Debbie darling,' she tells me over and over again. Isn't that strange? My mother is Jewish and my father Catholic, and I keep thinking it must have something to do with her Jewish beliefs. I really don't know. I keep mulling over what she could mean. My house is always clean, so it doesn't make any sense."

"This seems like an important dream, and she is definitely communicating something to you." I feel a flood of motherly love pour over me and my eyes mist with tears. "Oh Debbie, she loves you very much. I'm certainly not a medium, but the love you both share is very present right now. I feel a bit like I do when I'm with my own darling daughter, Beryl. But about your house … what house? Do you have several?"

"Nope, just one. But I have a spiritual streak in me and what keeps coming up is 'the house of the Lord.'"

"How fascinating, Debbie. Really, it's fascinating because the work we're doing here is internal work. I frequently say to clients, 'Let's get your house in order.' In a way, your body *is* the Lord's house, because you are part of creation. The waves on the ocean are not separate from the ocean; they *are* the ocean. Does that ring any bells?"

Debbie's eyes mist and she breaks into a sob. "My mother used to tell me all the time, 'Debbie, let's get your house in order and you'll get well,' but I forgot. Yes, my body is my true house … holding my spirit."

> *Postpartum depression should not be treated with antidepressants! Instead, missing hormones should be replaced.*

"I agree! Your body houses your precious spirit or soul. But what do you feel needs to be cleaned up in your body? What is so messy in this house of yours?"

She glances up at the ceiling. "I'm on these antidepressants, which aren't helping—and I eat sugar nonstop, drink about ten sodas a day, and I'm overweight. Dirty house, wow! Can any of these things cause depression?"

"A resounding YES! All of them can, but there is more, because your blood tests show that your estrogen is quite low. You're forty-two, right?"

"I turned forty-three two weeks ago." Debbie sighs.

"Happy birthday! But let's go back to when your depression began, which was triggered by having a baby. After we give birth our estrogen levels plummet and so can our thyroid hormones, and both cause postpartum depression. This etiology of depression shouldn't be treated with antidepressants. Instead, postpartum depression should be treated by replacing those missing hormones. Debbie, this is a no brainer. Your estrogen levels are really low now, and your testosterone is low too. Your results indicate that either a bit of perimenopause is creeping in or else you never really recovered your estrogen after your last childbirth. Regardless of the cause, beginning to use a bit of bioidentical estrogen and testosterone right away will really help."

Debbie's eyes light up. "I will—right now! I can't wait, but what about the thyroid?"

"It looks okay, but I want you to begin taking iodine to help your thyroid function more efficiently. Depression stems from so many different causes. It is always multifactorial, and it's our job to uncover each cause. Tell me about your kids and how all that is going."

"Well, they're older now and they're great. They really don't need me much except to drive them places, but even that is coming to an end now that they're seventeen and fifteen. My daughter is off to college in a year, and my son is a sports fanatic. My husband is dealing with all that and loves it."

"What about your life now that your mother career is winding down? What are your dreams for the next sixty years?

"Oh, God … sixty years? That's a long time. I don't know. I just don't know, and that's one of the reasons I keep feeling depressed. I got my MBA from UCLA and I had all kinds of plans, but being a mother put a stop to all that, especially when I started getting so depressed. Some nights I feel I can barely prepare dinner."

"Well, there is no doubt your low estrogen and testosterone derailed you, but your own life's journey is just as important as your children's. The transition from mother to Self is a profound one, and it's fraught with deep valleys and also many unexpected joys. Our Center's Path of Fulfillment helps our clients with important life transitions exactly like yours."

Debbie's face reflects vulnerability and love. I see her mother shining through. "Great! I'll do it. I have *got* to do it. I have lots more living to do, if only I can stop feeling so depressed. But you're right, feeling alone and not being part of life's excitement is depressing. I need to be the person I was meant to be before all this started. I have wasted so much time … It's all my fault."

I shake my head. "Deb, it is *not* your fault. It's the doctor's fault who missed what was really happening to you."

(I privately confess to myself that at times I also have been off the mark. A great deal of intense listening is required for a physician to track a problem to its root cause. Doctors need to be open to new ideas just as much as the IT industry must embrace new innovations.)

I recently spoke to a doctor friend of mine who showed me a Merck's Manual from 1918, which is one of the best manuals published each year to help doctors stay up on the most current treatments. In that 1918 edition there wasn't a single mention of antibiotics, hormones, or X-rays! The whole manual was about herbs and poisons. *And that was less than 100 years ago.* We knew nothing about current therapies, and today we know only a fraction of what we'll know in another hundred years. That realization keeps me humble and open-minded.

> *A great deal of intense listening is required for a physician to track a problem to its root cause.*

I think about how the medical community initially rejected the ideas and ridiculed the work of doctors who have pioneered groundbreaking treatments. From incubators for premature babies, washing one's hands before doing a delivery, to recognizing viruses as a cause of cancer, these and many other valuable medical contributions were at first rejected.

One of my dear friends, Bruce Hendricks, who was the CEO of Imation and Memorex, died a few years ago of a brain tumor. He used to tell me that he needed to live in order to help the medical field update itself. He said that if he ran his company the way the medical field operated he would be out of business in a month. He didn't live long enough to write his book and help transform our industry, but I agree with him 100 percent. And so I ask you this: Would you purchase a computer that is five years old? It is very unlikely, but if you were to, you'd know it was pretty outdated. New information in the medical field takes twenty-five years to become the "standard of care," which is like buying a twenty-five-year-old computer and acting like it's the hottest new item. So much death and suffering happens due to doctors following outdated information. In a hundred years we'll laugh (or cry) at the methods we use in medicine today. It's vital that physicians keep up with the progress being made in the medical field.

I smile at Debbie. "Your doctors just didn't understand about the root causes of postpartum depression. Initially, I didn't know it was caused by low estrogen or low thyroid either. But when I started measuring my depressed patients' hormone levels during my first few years of practice, I found their levels to be identical to those of my menopausal patients and immediately recognized a way to help them."

Debbie's face floods with relief. Her eyes scrunch up. "I have always been fascinated about technological advances and how information is lost and transmitted over the years. Maybe I can take up Bruce's mission and help with that."

I offer her a huge smile. We all must band together to help the world become a better place, and that mission would be a fascinating one. "Great, Deb! I would love to see you transform our field, so let's get you stronger first. We need to treat two more causes of your depression. Your blood sugar is quite high, and your sunshine hormone, D3, is very low—only fifteen, when it should be sixty-five to a hundred. Do you take a D3 supplement?"

Deborah shakes her head. "No one has ever checked my level before, so I didn't know I needed to take it."

"It's okay. We'll correct that right away to help with your depression, as well as decrease your risk of breast and colon cancer. We also want to clean up your diet. A good detox and some lifestyle changes will help you attain that really clean house."

Debbie looks down at her lap, then lifts her head momentarily to look into my eyes. "I don't know what to say. I've been chasing this depression problem for fifteen years, and maybe now that I finally have hope I'm a bit afraid I'll fail again. Do you really think all these suggestions will help? Really?"

I touch Deborah's knee and smile. "I'm not going to leave you alone in this. I can't let you fail. Your problems aren't hard to correct. Even if we aren't able to eradicate all your symptoms entirely, you will still feel a whole lot better. The rule is that with any low or missing hormone, we bring the numbers back to ideal, youthful levels. For example, your D3 level can be corrected by taking 10,000 IU of D3 a day. A small amount of estrogen cream will resolve your low estrogen problem, and a dab of natural testosterone cream will help with your depression and confidence. An iodine supplement and a small amount of thyroid hormone will also improve the way you feel. No wonder you're depressed! But you mentioned your diet is pretty bad too, didn't you? And what about exercise?"

> *"A high blood sugar level and a lack of nutrient absorption both cause depression."*

"I confess, my diet is really terrible, and I'm too depressed to exercise. I crave sugar and carbs all the time. I eat lots of pasta, bread and desserts. I just can't stop myself, probably because I'm so depressed."

"A high blood sugar level and a lack of nutrient absorption both cause depression," I tell her. "We need to clean up that diet of yours and get you on digestive enzymes, which will help you absorb your nutrients so much better. Our naturopaths will work with you next to get things sorted out with your diet and exercise."

Debbie smiles and I see some resolve coming back to her.

"So, let's bring this all together, okay? Your depression comes from having low thyroid that began during your pregnancy. Your baby took all your iodine for herself, which caused your own thyroid hormone to become depleted. Your estrogen was low after your delivery, which was missed, and you were put on antidepressants that didn't treat the root causes of your depression. This caused you to feel exhausted and gain weight, which added to your depression. The antidepressants also killed your libido. Your estrogen and testosterone are both low, and your D3 is low because you don't get much sun exposure. Your diet is a problem, and so is the NutraSweet in your sodas—both of which cause depression. And last but not least, you have a need to find yourself and your new Life Mission."

With tears in her eyes, Debbie pulls back her shoulders as she raises her eyes to look into mine. "Thank you, Prudence. I feel hopeful now that we're going to try something different. No one has ever taken an approach even close to this and I certainly want to try it. What about the antidepressants? Do I continue taking them?"

"No! Let's begin the weaning process today, but we need to go very slowly. You're on 150 mg, isn't that right?"

"Right, and I want to come off them. They aren't helping me."

"Taking you off them will be part of our house cleaning. No more clutter! I'll write a prescription for 100 mg a day. I also want you to start taking a supplement I formulated called Bliss, a unique combination of herbs and other supplements that act as a natural antidepressant. It will cause you to feel quite happy naturally by supporting your brain's own neurotransmitters and hormones, and will also help you wean off the Zoloft. In a month we'll lower you to 75 mg of Zoloft, and then very slowly take you off completely over the next few months. You've taken antidepressants for so many years that we need to go very slowly. Does this sound okay?"

Debbie's face beams with life. "Yes, more than okay—perfect, really. I have been trying to get off them but my doctor didn't have any other solutions for my depression."

"I also feel a nutrient IV or 'push' would be an excellent choice to jumpstart you out of depression. Would you like our Naturopathic doctor to put together a combination for you?"

"I would love that!" She stops and scrunches up her face as she continues. "And I have a feeling that a whole new life is waiting for me. How do I get involved in the Path of Fulfillment program?"

"We publish the evening events on our website and send out notices. I have many clients who break the mold of who they have been to become completely new people with new interests, careers, friends and places to live. We humans are capable of extraordinary life transitions. I call this 'Soul Health.' I'll give you a flyer for your notebook. I just want to say before you leave that all this takes a bit of time. Would you give me three or four months to help you get the best results?"

"Sure, Prudence. I understand my depression wasn't created in a month, so it will take time to resolve."

"Thanks, Deb. It takes time to get the hormones into your body and help you begin to make your own 'feel good' hormones. We need to rebuild and restore you back to your healthy, joyful self."

I am hopeful she will begin to feel some relief in the first month, but I don't want her to become discouraged if it takes a few months. Deb and I have had a long dialogue, and at the end she is ready to meet the rest of her team. I hug her warmly as she leaves the room and notice that she has a little energy in her step, which she didn't have when she first came in.

Her nutrition program is easily set up to include lots of greens and healthy protein, digestive enzymes with her meals, and sparkling water with lime rather than sodas—and, of course, no sugar. She is given a stool kit to see if she has parasites or problems with her digestive tract. We will review the results at her next meeting.

Debbie returns to see me in one month. She smiles and actually laughs. "Prudence, I don't know what's happening to me! I really can't believe it. I have so much more energy than I used to, and I'm not staying in bed nearly as much as before. I've been doing three clicks of estrogen, just like you told me, and my depression is not nearly as bad."

I review Debbie's labs and see that her estrogen and testosterone levels are in the ideal range but her thyroid didn't respond as well to iodine as I had hoped, so I prescribe one grain of natural thyroid. Unfortunately, her stool results show she has H. Pylori and yeast, which has most likely been contributing to her depression and her inability to lose weight. Given her stool findings a dietary detox will not be enough. This is our naturopath's specialty and I imagine she will treat Debbie with herbs and a gut restoration protocol.

> *She is like a flower opening up into greater and greater beauty.*

Debbie has been very motivated to clean up her diet which will help her digestive system heal faster. She has opted to work with one of our mind-body practitioners who does Trilo Therapy. It was developed by Nissim Amon, a Zen master and my friend. In a dialogue, the practitioner talks with both the client's head and heart, which are usually not in agreement with each other. Either the head refuses to let the heart express herself, or the heart has somehow hijacked the head. In either case, inner turmoil and unhappiness arise. How will this conflicting inner chatter resolve itself? By the clarity of True Self—Observer—living at the center of all beings. It is tremendously effective work, and in only three sessions Debbie has much more clarity as to why she is unhappy and how to break herself out of habitual patterns, which cause depression.

Debbie tells me she also started the weekly meditations at the Center with Anil Chandwani and has elected to work with him concerning what's missing in her life. She feels so much happier and excited with her mentoring and tells me she is cooking up a new life for herself.

We spend a few minutes going over what Debbie has learned about herself and some of the options she has been thinking about for her future. She is like a flower opening up into greater and greater beauty. Before leaving, we give her a heavy metal kit to see if she has mercury, lead, or other heavy metal toxicity—all of which are known causes of depression.

Debbie returns in three months for her consult and she is exploding with energy. She is down to just 25 mg of Zoloft each day, and we agree to decrease her to half a pill and then come off completely in three weeks. Her thyroid is completely normal after taking thyroid supplementation and her estrogen and testosterone levels are still normal. She has lost fifteen pounds and her sex drive is picking up due to her testosterone use and decreased Zoloft. She is more involved with her kids and is starting a new business with a few of her mom friends who also left their careers when they became mothers. When I ask Debbie about it her face lights up.

> "If depression ever hovers near me, which it almost never does, I see it as a cloud floating by in the sky. Maybe it'll rain a bit, or maybe the sun will shine. It's okay to let my emotions flow."

"Well, I am actually involved in helping people with their depression online. I am starting with that, and then I'll keep adding the most up-to-date information on a number of medical diseases. One of my partners was a medical researcher before she had kids, and I understand the technology part of this … we already launched. I am super into the mind-body aspect of health. I now meditate, thanks to Anil and also the Mentors Channel programs. It's changing my life and has helped with my depression. If depression ever hovers near me, which it almost never does, I see it as a cloud floating by in the sky. Maybe it'll rain a bit, or maybe the sun will shine. It's okay to let my emotions flow. But really, I am not depressed now. I have no time!" She laughs and asks if I can prescribe a bit more time for her because she's too busy.

"Sure, honey!" I whip out my pad and write a prescription for "Timeless creation, unending joy." We exchange smiles and my heart swells as I give Debbie a goodbye hug. She is a dear one and I see her as a bright light going back into the world, bringing light and love to those she touches.

Six months have gone by and I haven't heard from Debbie. I wonder if she is okay, so I ask my nurse to drop her an email and get this response in return:

Dear Prudence,

I am so embarrassed that I haven't written or come in, but I am happy to say that I am not feeling badly at all. In fact, I can't believe what is happening to me. I moved to Israel to reconnect to my roots. I think my mother wanted me to do this as part of my house cleaning. I love it! My husband has a great job here and the kids are all in school. They are not fluent in Hebrew yet, but they are better than I am! I have a new life, a new house, and am moving full speed ahead with all the work I did at the Center. I am volunteering with Mentors Channel and am also studying Trilo Therapy with Nissim to be a practitioner. I am learning a lot. I realized I like working with people and think I'll start teaching English to adults and somehow combine it with meditation.

I'll stay on top of my hormones, promise. Can I do a phone consult in a few months? My blessings to everyone at the Center.

Shalom,

Debbie Cohen

I am relieved and joyful. Her joy is mine. We are all one!

Takeaway:

Depression has various root causes including low estrogen due to menopause, perimenopause, the birth control pill, and being postpartum. It is also caused by low thyroid hormones and low adrenal stress hormones, as well as low D3, the sunshine hormone. Balancing your hormones is paramount! Toxicity from environmental pollutants causes depression by overwhelming the liver's ability to detoxify. Gut imbalances and toxicity also play a role. Diet sodas specifically cause depression, and so can food we're intolerant or allergic to. Challenging life transitions add to depression, especially the mid-life transitions women face when their children begin to leave the house or their careers become less interesting.

My prescription for depression and anxiety:

- Balance your estrogen, thyroid, adrenal hormones and D3 with bioidentical hormones.

- Take Biodine (Body Software): 1 capsule daily to help your thyroid gland function better.

- Eat a healthy diet filled with nutritious super food and limit or eliminate gluten, sugar, corn and soy.

- Sleep deeply for 8 hours; take Sweet Sleep (Body Software): 1-2 capsules at sleep as needed.

- Discontinue the birth control pill and use a non-hormonal method such as the Paraguard IUD, condoms or a diaphragm.

- Bliss (Body Software): take 1-2 capsules each day.

- Identify and reduce stress by using the WellBe bracelet.

- Engage in some form of physical activity daily.

- Seek help from a skilled therapist.

- Consider a transformational program such as Landmark Worldwide or Ger Lyons' Core & Cellular Transformation.

- Work with a mentor to help identify your life goals and implement them.

- Do Doron Libshtein's *Walk your Path* program located on mentorschannel.com.

- Meditate and/or establish a practice like Chi Gong or yoga.

- Create a community of friends and meet with them to have dinners, celebrations, and support.

- Be a Johnny Appleseed and plant love everywhere. It will grow and flourish.

Chapter 7

Exhaustion and Fatigue

"I am so tired, I just can't get out of bed some days," Antonia moans. "I used to have all the energy in the world without any down time. I can't even tell you how much I used to do, but now … I don't even recognize the person I have become."

Antonia has flown in from Italy, full of despair. She comes from Rome where several of her friends who are my patients have "forced" her to come for a consult. I am moved by the effort she has made, an indicator of the pain she's in.

"Antonia," I respond, reaching out to touch her with a light gesture, "how did this start? How long have you been feeling this way?"

"Well, I have always had such enormous energy. I'm only forty-two and for most of my life I've had the energy of three people. People always told me, 'Antonia, we can't keep up with you! You are a whirlwind and can do anything!' But now I can barely get out of bed. Yes, of course I do what needs to be done, but I fake it. I go to the store and spend time with my kids, but nothing more than that. I can't go out with my friends or do dinner parties like

I used to, or really do any of the things I used to love doing. I simply don't have the energy." She hangs her head and sighs.

"It started two years ago after my father died suddenly. He was my dearest friend, and lived with me, my husband and our children. I went looking for him that day because he was not up making his usual espresso. I checked his room and then went out to the orchard. I found him there, crumpled, with an expression of pain on his face. He always walked, but he told me he had been experiencing a bit of fatigue the prior few weeks. Dr. Hall, he had a massive heart attack. I never realized he was sick because I was fooled by his youthful, enthusiastic manner so never made him go to the doctor. If I had he might still be alive. We all went into tremendous mourning. Right after that I got quite tired and started needing more sleep. I recovered after a few months but then, for no apparent reason, this downward spiral began. Each week I had to force myself more and more to get up. Little by little I gave up my activities until I became a shell of who I used to be. When people ask how I am doing I smile and laugh like I always used to, but inside I'm not laughing. I'm trying to stop myself from crying, because I know I'm not doing well. I am not well at all, and I'm afraid something is very wrong. Could I have the same health issue my father did? I'm so worried."

> *Fatigue stems from so many different causes, with adrenal exhaustion being the most prominent source.*

My heart fills with compassion for this lovely lady. "Have you seen doctors in Italy? What do they tell you? Fatigue can be caused by a wide variety of issues."

"I saw a cardiologist because of my dad's condition and he said I am as healthy as a child. My cholesterol is 148 and I have no plaque in my arteries. My regular doctor did a cancer work up. My colon, uterus, ovaries and breasts are fine. My blood work is perfect. The neurologist said I don't have a brain tumor. They finally said I might have chronic fatigue and checked me for the Epstein Barr and mono viruses. I was negative for both, so they ended up telling me I am okay.

She pauses and slumps her shoulders. "Can you believe it? I can't get out of bed, but they tell me everything is okay. But I am *not* okay at all. I mean, how can there be nothing wrong when I feel this way? And if there is really nothing wrong, then I am in big trouble because I can't live like this—I have become a nothing."

I feel Antonia's urgency and go into high gear. Fatigue is one of the most common problems I am presented with and it is always a complex issue. It stems from so many different causes, with adrenal exhaustion being the most prominent source. I sit back to hear more about Antonia's fatigue, looking for more telltale symptoms of stress.

"So, Antonia," I probe, "if ten is the most energy you've ever had and zero the least, what level is your energy when you wake up?"

She is quiet and I sense her mind at work. "Well, if zero is the least energy I could have, I am a one or two out of ten when I wake up in the morning."

"That's pretty tired," I sympathize. "What about at noon?"

"I peak with my energy around ten in the morning with a four out of ten, probably because I have had several espressos, and then by lunch time I am a three out of ten. After three in the afternoon I am a zero or one. I just can't get off the couch."

"Poor Antonia! That is really tired. What about feelings of depression or panic?"

"Yes, I feel nervous all the time and am down and kind of sad for no reason. Initially, I was depressed because of my dad's death and cried all the time. Then I started feeling panicky and needed to stop driving. I'm now driving again but am so fearful. I have constant internal worries and anxiety." Her eyes plead with me for help.

"Do you want to tell me more about it?" I encourage.

She hesitates and then blurts it out, "I'm afraid my husband will leave me. He is ten years older than I, but a bundle of energy. He runs, hikes, and works ten hours a day and he's never tired! All I do is stay in bed. How often can I refuse to make love because I am too tired, or stay home when he goes out to dinner? I am his young wife so I try and keep this condition to myself. I can't really tell him how bad it is. It's not right to burden him." She bursts into tears of grief, clasping her knees with her arms, rocking herself. I reach over to cradle her shoulders and help her rock away some of the pain.

When she is calmer I share her blood work with her. "Antonia, many things cause fatigue. One of your problems is right here in black and white: You have adrenal deficiency. All four of your adrenal hormones are very low. I mean crashed and collapsed values, which is quite concerning. Your adrenal hormones come from your adrenal glands, which are located on top of your kidneys. When you experience a shock or stress, large amounts of hormones are released to manage the stress. Having three children, your dad's sudden death, your sleeplessness and emotional issues—these things all tax the glands and use up your hormones. Sometimes we just can't reintroduce the hormones fast enough. Symptoms of adrenal deficiency are fatigue, which is usually worse in the afternoon, as well as depression, panic or anxiety, hair loss, food cravings and a low sex drive. Does this sound like you?"

"Absolutely!" Antonia replies. "My dad's death was the most traumatic event I have ever experienced, but the stress actually started before that. You know men—especially Italian men." She tosses her head back. "I can tell you this because you are a woman, so I already know you will understand. Four years ago I found out my husband was having an affair. I was so upset I wanted to leave him but—I love him. He is a good man and I saw that my rage wouldn't help our marriage so I stuffed it down inside me and suffered alone. I also vowed to myself to be everything for him, which helped renew our marriage. I started being the fun person

> When you experience a shock or stress, large amounts of hormones are released to manage the stress.

I was before the kids, became super loving again, and he soon gave up his other lover. But the stress was awful. I had to carry the humiliation alone. He's the type of person who never admits he is wrong so we couldn't go into therapy together."

We sit silently for a few minutes and I think about my first marriage to a French-Spanish aristocrat. I was living in France at the time, and while affairs are accepted as "normal" in that society, I was a young bride who never imagined it could happen in my relationship. When I found out after six years of marriage that he had engaged in a few hundred affairs it shattered my heart. It also made me feel alone and I began to adopt a kind of emotional bravado. I told myself that my happiness shouldn't need to come from another person; it was 100 percent my job to make myself happy. In reality, I was actually not that strong—I was dealing with trauma. As I matured over the years I realized that real courage came from my ability to love and trust. However, when I left that marriage I was deep into my medical studies and felt more sure of myself and my destiny.

I nod my head. "I do understand, Antonia, and I know the stress this puts on our bodies, what with the enormous heartache and constant vigilance it takes to overcome such a thing. You are not alone. I have certainly experienced it and so have many other women. This factor, along with your pregnancies, raising young children, and your dad's death have all contributed to a state of adrenal deficiency—in your case—burnout." I show Antonia her lab values, which are in the bottom 5 percent when compared to ideal values.

> *"Your pregnancies, raising young children, and your dad's death have all contributed to a state of adrenal deficiency—in your case—burnout."*

Antonia shakes her head, her eyes full of sadness. "It's all true. I would have tried to handle things better but the stress was just overwhelming. So now what is there to do? It seems pretty hopeless with these low levels."

I offer an encouraging smile. "Antonia, we can fix this! It will take time, perhaps up to six months, but truly you will get your energy back. First, we need to augment all four of your adrenal hormones with natural bioidentical hormones. I have compounded a supplement called Super Adrenal, which has almost everything you need and is a real miracle. I used to prescribe four different adrenal supplements, but I combined them all into this one potent combination. Start taking one capsule each morning, along with one pill of natural cortisol in the morning, at lunch, and the late afternoon. This natural hormone is safe and bioidentical to your own hormone that is so low. The goal is to take you off everything once your adrenals heal, but for now these supplements are lifesavers—they are like a cast for a broken leg. Also, you need to sleep well at night. With adrenal fatigue, what little energy you do have often comes at night. Are you finding it harder to sleep?"

> *"We call this 'wired and tired,' when depleted adrenal glands begin to produce more hormones at night."*

Antonia's eyes grow wide. "Absolutely, I have a surge of energy around ten o'clock at night. I go from exhaustion to agitation, and then I can't sleep. I'm exhausted, but also restless and edgy. If I stay up, the next day my energy level is a zero out of ten all day. There's not even a glimmer of hope."

"When depleted adrenal glands begin to produce more hormones at night, we call this 'wired and tired.' An essential part of your treatment will be to restore your adrenal glands so you sleep deeply nine or more hours a day—not just resting or fighting to stay awake. Do you see this bracelet I'm wearing? It's called the WellBe and monitors my stress continuously throughout the day.

I want you to get one so you can identify when you're stressed and have a solution right then and there. When I started wearing mine I saw that throughout the day my stress was at 85 percent. I was headed for problems but have now been able to keep my stress level in the healthy range. I want you to wear one. Would that be okay?"

"Sure Dr. Hall, absolutely."

"Great! I am happy about that. I'd also like to prescribe Sweet Sleep."

"Yes, oh yes, I will do everything you say, Dr. Hall. I have to overcome this fatigued state."

"Antonia, please call me Prudence, like everyone else does."

She smiles. "Italian doctors are not like that. They want to be called 'doctor.'"

I return her smile. "Well, I am pretty sure of my knowledge, so I don't actually need the encouragement of the title." We both giggle at this feminine way of approaching each other. Women need relatedness, and that includes me.

I look further down her chart. "I see another cause of fatigue. Are you ever cold, constipated or experiencing hair loss?"

She doesn't miss a beat. "You're asking about my thyroid, aren't you? Well, I thought for sure I was low but all my doctors tell me my thyroid is fine."

I glance at her thyroid blood work and immediately see that her blood tests, although "normal," are not ideal. On her Thyroflex questionnaire she scores fifty-seven symptoms of low thyroid. That is a lot! Her Thyroflex reflex result is quite elevated, indicating a 95 percent likelihood that she has a thyroid deficiency.

"Bingo," I say triumphantly. "One for the home team. Antonia, you know more about diagnosing thyroid disease than your doctors. You definitely have a low functioning (hypothyroid) gland." I show her the results and she shakes her head in disbelief.

> *We begin with the basic ABC's to make sure we leave nothing to chance.*

"I knew it! I just knew it. I can't believe it was missed."

"I detest it when this happens, Antonia." I touch her hand. "I regret that you suffered for so long without help and we will correct this problem now. Let's start you on a course of iodine, a natural mineral needed for thyroid hormone production. So many patients have low iodine levels, especially women who have had children. The baby's need for iodine depletes mom's own stores. I'd also like to prescribe some natural thyroid hormones. You've read the books and understand the different types of thyroid replacement, and for your case I would like to use a natural T3-T4 combination. What do you think?"

Antonia gives me a weak, hopeful smile. "More than okay. This is now my lifeline."

I peruse the rest of Antonia's blood work. She is not perimenopausal or menopausal, even given my very subtle ways of diagnosing these early stages of decline. Neither does she have high blood sugar or much cellular damage due to sugar. This is great, because a damaged metabolism from insulin resistance or diabetes causes tremendous fatigue. Her hematocrit is also excellent. She is not anemic. Perhaps she is dealing with exposure to a virus like Lyme or one of the other fatigue viruses like Epstein Barr. Or maybe she has mercury, lead, mold, or other toxic exposures. She could have gut dysfunction (digestive problems), which so many people suffer from, or a parasite that causes fatigue. I glance at her questionnaire and it is absent of any gut symptoms. With Antonia, we begin with the basic ABC's to make sure we leave nothing to chance. Having dealt with literally thousands of fatigue cases, doing the most basic things often results in a huge energy payoff.

Antonia is relieved by my proposed plan of action. I love educated patients! This health game we all play is definitely a team sport. Before our consult closes, I add a sophisticated cellular energy supplement called Cellular Radiance because it will help the mitochondria of her cells (the energy power plants) create more energy. Treating fatigue is both an inside and outside job.

"So," I continue, "our treatment so far is sleep, natural hormones, and definitely a healthy diet. Certain grain and dairy-rich diets are inflammatory, causing fatigue and allergies. Too much or too little exercise stresses the adrenals and so does internal emotional conflict. An important treatment will be a series of IV nutrient infusions or 'pushes' to help restore your adrenal glands." I glance at Antonia and can tell she fully understands what I'm saying. "I'd like you to take one infusion week while you're in the United States. Your next appointment is with our naturopath to evaluate your digestive health and toxic metals, and then with our mind-body specialist who will work with you on healing from past trauma. How does this sound?"

She smiles with delight and we hug warmly. I feel such affection and respect for this courageous soul. We walk out of my office, where our naturopath greets her. Antonia needs a comprehensive approach to turn fatigue into power, passion and abundant energy.

> *Testosterone comes from the adrenal gland as well as from the ovaries, and Antonia's value is almost zero.*

I think about many of the patients I have treated for fatigue over the years and the difficult times when I've been exhausted myself. When I was in medical school the stresses of long, sleepless nights and so many sick patients almost crushed me. My first divorce was also very difficult and when my former husband later died in a plane crash—long after we had become close friends—I started to feel shaky and sick. Bringing his ashes back to his heartbroken parents, whom I loved very much, and dealing with my loss as well caused my adrenal glands to collapse. I spoke of this in another chapter, so suffice it to say that learning to deal with stress as well as avoiding new stress helped restore my energy. Our adrenal program helps patients who suffer as I did to find new inner peace, regain their energy and resolve the pain of exhaustion. Disconnecting from the past is a good place to begin emotionally because it frees us to be our true selves and loving ambassadors to the world.

Antonia's trip to the United States will end in three weeks, so we put her into an accelerated mode of two IV infusions per week, more detox treatments with our naturopath, and two good lymph massages. She meets with our nurse practitioner,

Stephanie, who is an ace with aesthetic skin rejuvenation, doing a combination SkinFinity (radio frequency) and PRP treatment. By the time Antonia is ready to leave, she feels much better about her appearance, and is feeling 10 to 15 percent better.

⚬

In three weeks, I call Antonia in Rome and ask how she's doing.

"Better!" I hear the delight in her voice. "I'm probably feeling better—maybe 25 percent, and it feels like a flame of energy is starting."

She is still unsure because of jet lag, but it feels like something important is happening. I tell her to begin taking two Super Adrenals each day and to increase the natural thyroid to one-and-a-half pills. I've received her testosterone level results from her first visit, and it is extremely low. Testosterone comes from the adrenal gland as well as from the ovaries, and her value is almost zero. We agree to add a dose of natural testosterone cream to Antonia's program, as this will help build muscle and self-confidence along with augmenting her low libido. Healthy testosterone levels are critical for energy.

⚬

Three weeks later I Skype with Antonia who is now in Sardinia on vacation. I rejoice when she tells me she is feeling considerably better.

"Prudence, I can't believe this. You told me this would take

Antonia says, "I think we are experiencing more closeness because I am sharing my emotions with him rather than keeping this all to myself."

six months but I am really feeling better! I don't stay in bed like I used to. I take a long nap but I don't feel I'm dying like I did before. The testosterone cream is great and I have made love with my husband a few times. He is acting really sweet. I think we are experiencing more closeness because I am sharing my emotions with him rather than keeping this all to myself."

Antonia pushes a wisp of jet black hair away from her eyes and continues. "I love my WellBe and am shocked by how stressed I am. I listen to the Mind Travel music on the WellBe non stop and I have also gone to Mentors Channel to learn more about meditation. In one of the audio downloads I heard loud and clear: 'I want for you what you want for you.' Marco told me he had felt very lonely when I wouldn't share what was going on with me. I could hardly talk to him before because of my shame at being so sick and his past betrayal. Now that doesn't feel so important. I was also helped by a mentor saying, 'Nothing happens *to* me; it happens *for* me.' I think that's right and I feel so much more powerful—and sexy."

Toxic levels of mercury cause quite pronounced fatigue.

She gives me the biggest smile and I study her carefully. I celebrate Antonia's victories with her and sit back to hear more of her life-realizations. I think she is a teacher at heart and I tell her that.

"Well, from suffering comes power, passion and purpose, right? Isn't that what you told me the first day I met you?" Antonia gives me a coy grin.

This time I'm the one who laughs! "Why, yes, maestro-teacher," then add more seriously, "Antonia, you are better and you will continue to improve, but we need to make sure we are treating *all* your causes of fatigue. How much better do you think you are? What percentage?"

"Well," she bites her lower lip and sucks her breath in. "I guess about 40 percent. But it feels like a new life. Really, I know I'm not dying now."

"Good, I am so glad, but we need to treat something else. I have your toxic metal urine test back and I'm sorry to say your mercury is sky high. It is in the danger zone, which is one reason your thyroid is low. Toxic levels of mercury cause quite pronounced fatigue."

> *We can detoxify to help the mercury leave the body with a supplement called DMSA, and also vitamin C, chlorella and cilantro.*

I see shock spread over Antonia's face. "Mercury? That's terrible. I have read all about it. Where is it coming from?"

"Unfortunately, it mainly comes from eating fish, the environment, dental amalgams, or perhaps from vaccines that use mercury as a preservative. How are your teeth, Antonia?"

"Terrible!" her response leaps off the screen. "Just terrible. I had mercury fillings when I was ten and they are starting to fall out. I have about twelve of them so they could be leaking."

"Yes, they could be. I'd like you to go to a dentist to have them checked, but choose a dentist who is holistic in his approach.

When removing them, he needs to use all precautions to avoid spreading the mercury. We can detoxify to help the mercury leave the body with a supplement called DMSA, and also vitamin C, chlorella and cilantro. But really, Antonia, you mustn't eat fish. That's so unfortunate but seafood is toxic these days."

"If it helps me regain my health I'll stop eating fish altogether. No problem." I see the determination in her eyes. "Can you send me the vitamin C and detox items? I want to get started."

"Of course. We'll send them right out. Your adrenal hormones are improving but I want to give you a stronger adrenal mixture called Mega Adrenal. It has 15 mg of DHEA and a larger amount of pregnenolone in it plus other natural herbs. Just take one of them and finish up your Super Adrenal by taking three each morning. Also take two of the cortisol each morning and one in the afternoon. You are soaking this up!" Antonia laughs and I feel new levity in her manner. "Have a wonderful vacation, dear wonder woman, and I hope you get to make love in lots of fun places. After all, you are Italian!"

> *Antonia has become one of the wise women who, through the portal of pain, retrieved her vital self.*

Antonia and I talk in another month and she is much better. She has resumed 80 percent of her prior activities and tells me she has found her laughing nature again. She and Marco are doing great and with her Shakti back she tells me his eyes are looking for hers like they used to. We make adjustments in her program and she tells me she will be returning to California to do some of the deeper heavy metal detoxes we had discussed. Her fillings have all been replaced with nontoxic material and she wants another kit to measure the levels. This is great news because treating toxicity will not only give her more energy,

> *Treating toxicity will not only give her more energy, but will also decrease her risk of cancer and chronic diseases.*

it will also decrease her risk of cancer and chronic diseases. We laugh, talk a few more minutes and then sign off.

Fast forward ten years to another Skype appointment with Antonia. When we hang up I sit quietly thinking about her transformation out of crippling exhaustion to being fully functional, energetic and happy. It was an amazing journey: exhausted adrenals, low thyroid, heavy metal toxicity, and emotional pain. She had so many causes of her fatigue. We have stayed in contact for more than ten years and it is always a wonderful celebration when we talk. Antonia has become one of the wise women who, through the portal of pain, retrieved her vital self. After she became well and strong she studied herbal medicine and became an herbal specialist. She opened a practice combining mind-body medicine and was recently interviewed by the biggest newspaper in Rome. Her marriage is vital and she has grown into an emotionally sophisticated communicator. What a privilege to have helped her in her time of need. I continue to be one of her mentors, and she has been one of mine.

> *While in this cocoon phase, I realized I was actually quite traumatized by all the pain I had been witnessing.*

Fly high and strong dear Antonia, on your journey from Me, to We, to One.

I think back to my own journey with the problem of fatigue. When I was in my gynecology residency program at USC, we were taught to pretty much ignore ourselves and "show up" no matter what happened. I was working more than eighty hours a week and, after several years, became quite ill. I started losing my hair, became depressed, and gained weight. I couldn't think as clearly as I once did and became worried about having something seriously wrong with my brain. One of my friends, a neurology resident, offered to help. When his workup was done, he said he had bad news: I had an untreatable disease called "gynecology residency." I stared at him blankly and then we both started laughing so hard we were literally howling. When we finally were too exhausted to laugh any more we figured out all the nutrients I needed for nutrient drips. I did these two or three times a week and began to feel better. When my vacation finally arrived, I stayed in bed twenty-four hours a day for the first two weeks. I literally didn't leave the bed—I just read and slept. I couldn't believe how much better I felt. While in this cocoon phase I realized I was actually quite traumatized by all the pain I had been witnessing. My decision to journal about it was the start of my "soul health."

> *I saw that by acknowledging how I felt, many of the fears I had been suppressing disappeared.*

I saw that by acknowledging how I felt many of the fears I had been suppressing disappeared. I witnessed how afraid I was of dying. I was also afraid of being destitute or infertile. I imagined the pain of delivering all my patients' babies while failing to have any of my own. The list went on and on. I decided I needed to bring more peace into my thoughts so I started meditating. Meditation slowly reconnected me to my source of inner love and I felt moments of bliss as my fears lifted. I started using meditation and energetic medicine for my own healing, and I saw that when I was connected I didn't experience life in such an exhausting manner. Our thoughts really do matter! Healing is an inside job. Health is not just an absence of disease, it is vitality, wisdom, passion and peace.

> *Healing is an inside job. Health is not just an absence of disease, it is vitality, wisdom, passion and peace.*

❧

My twenty-eight-year-old daughter Beryl interrupts my writing. "Morning Mom, hurry up! You have a patient." My three children are a source of constant joy to me, and it is so fun to have my daughter at the Center with me. I know it will only be for a few more months because, guess what? She has been accepted to Bastyr University to become a Naturopathic doctor, and what a wonderful one she will be! I am already scheming to woo her back to the clinic when she graduates.

> "You were born with potential. You were born
> with goodness and trust. You were born with
> ideals and dreams. You were born with greatness.
> You were born with wings. You are not meant
> for crawling, so don't. You have wings.

Learn to use them and fly."

—Rumi

Takeaway:

Fatigue and exhaustion have multiple etiologies: adrenal depletion, low thyroid states, low estrogen from the pill, menopause, perimenopause or the postpartum state. Toxicity is another frequently overlooked cause of fatigue, including toxicity from heavy metals, a toxic gut, and mold exposure. Lyme and Epstein-Barr are common culprits of fatigue, along with trauma and unfulfilled dreams, which often trigger depression and fatigue.

Supplements:

- Super Adrenal for women: 1-3 capsules depending on severity of fatigue (begin with 1 capsule)
- Mega Adrenal for men: 1-2 capsules for men (begin with 1 capsule)
- Cellular Radiance: 3 capsules per day
- Biodine: 1 capsule per day to help the thyroid function better
- Feminine Radiance: 1-3 capsules per day for women over age 35
- Restoring Digestive health with enzymes, probiotics, and parasite treatment
- IV nutrients for adrenal healing and cellular health
- WellBe bracelet for monitoring your stress

Chapter 8

Breast Cancer and Menopause

I meet Lauren on a rainy February day, the rain happily reminding me of the great Northwest where I lived as a child. I usher her into my consult room where she offers me a forced smile as she sits down. I look into her eyes searching for what she might need. I sense her reticent nature, so I start the conversation. "Lauren, I am so happy to meet you. Shall we share some tea together on this beautiful wet day and talk about your concerns?"

Lauren shifts her gaze to the edge of the window frame behind me. "I've traveled all night to come here and now that I'm meeting you, I really don't know why I came. I guess I just don't feel like myself. I'm fifty-two years old and work non-stop as a corporate attorney in a big firm. As the mother of two kids, I'm the only provider for the family since my divorce. While on the plane last night, I had a chance to think about my life. I love my children. They're sixteen and seventeen and they're great kids. Now that they're driving they need me less, and in a few years they'll both be away at college … so, I guess that's all okay.

"As for my job, I've definitely done contract work for too long so it's no longer very interesting. I just don't seem to have the same drive I used to have. But I was asking myself if these things

Radiant Again & Forever

could make my life feel so hard. It doesn't seem like much has changed but maybe *I've* changed because I no longer like my life. I've been going over and over this in my mind, asking myself, '*What's wrong? What's wrong?!*' I guess it boils down to this: I just can't believe this is all there is to life."

I listen to every word, sensing her fear and hopelessness. "It can feel pretty dark, can't it, Lauren? So many women are in various life crises when they come to me. You're at that perfect transition where it's important to evaluate your life and decide how to create more meaning and happiness. Our lives pass so quickly, that eighty years can feel like a flash. What about your physical symptoms? Do you feel energetic and strong?"

"Well." She lets out a deep breath. "I have hot flashes, can't sleep at night and am extremely tired. I can also be a total bitch. I get so irritated with my kids that I can't stand myself, and I am actually quite depressed. So I guess that's not feeling 'strong' at all. I feel pretty awful actually, and I've gained thirty-five pounds. I've done a lot of reading so I know I'm probably in premenopause, or do we say perimenopause? I still have regular periods but I haven't felt well for five or six years. The thing is, I don't want to take hormones and I know you are a hormone specialist. Maybe I shouldn't have come." She looks down at her hands and sighs.

> *The easiest ones to correct are your hormonal imbalances, so let's start with that.*

"Lauren, there are many issues to discuss. The easiest ones to correct are your hormonal imbalances so let's start with that. I have your lab results and I hope this isn't going to upset you, but your labs indicate you are deep into menopause. You probably went into perimenopause a few years before you started feeling so badly, and menopause two or three

> *Many women are shocked to be menopausal, with it traditionally being a secret, private transition.*

years ago." I open her patient notebook and show her the hormone graph and how low her hormones are. She gasps and puts her hands over her eyes, her chin quivering.

"I can't believe it! I know I am the right age but I still have my periods. How can this be?" She stifles a sob.

"Oh, Lauren, I'm so sorry this upsets you." Did you know that most women begin menopause between the ages of forty-five and forty-eight? It's happening earlier than it used to and many women are menopausal even at forty."

"Oh, no! I had no idea it could start so early. Dr. Hall, I feel so old and unattractive. I don't want anyone to know. It feels like no one will want me anymore."

"Dear, beautiful Lauren, look at yourself! You are so lovely! How can a lab result change that? But you are not alone in feeling this way. Many women are shocked to be menopausal, traditionally keeping it a secret, private transition. Most women tell me they are reluctant to share, even with other women. But why don't you believe in using bioidentical hormones? The data about them is so positive and women who use them feel amazing and actually live longer. Why are you so sure you don't want to take them?"

After a few moments Lauren shares her heart, her voice quivering. "Dr. Hall, I didn't put it on my information sheet, but I had breast cancer four years ago. I had radiation treatments and chemo because I had two positive lymph nodes. I just can't risk the cancer returning." She closes her eyes and rocks back and forth, clutching her arms around herself. "Now I am doubly unattractive—breast cancer *and* menopause. A double whammy!" Her eyes fill with tears. "The word *menopause* reminds me of my grandmother and her wrinkled skin, all her medications and that old-person smell. I don't want that! I really don't want that. Please help me, please! But I just can't risk taking anything that will put me at a higher risk for cancer again. I have to be here for my kids."

> *"It has been shown that natural progesterone actually prevents breast cancer, and the bioidentical estrogen either shows no increased risk of breast cancer or a slight decrease."*

I quietly wait before I respond. "First, please call me Prudence. We are getting into a serious conversation, and I want you to feel fully empowered." I smile at her. "Is that okay, counselor?" She smiles and nods. "Okay, so our common goal is to help you love your life and stay healthy and beautiful for many more years—and certainly to be here for your kids as long as possible."

"Oh yes, yes! I want to stay healthy and raise my kids and be a grandmother to my grandkids. There is no question that I'm willing to do whatever I can to stay alive and be healthy. Beautiful would be wonderful, too." She smiles as though telling a little joke.

I straighten up in my chair. "Okay, let's dive into this. Using hormones with patients who have had breast cancer is certainly controversial. I don't know how much you've learned, but it is widely believed by both doctors and patients alike that hormones cause breast cancer. This information came out of the Women's Health Initiative Study published in 2001. The study involved the use of synthetic, non-bioidentical hormones like Premarin and Provera. The study initially concluded that these synthetic hormones increased the incidence of breast cancer, with the synthetic progesterone called Provera being the major contributor to the increase. The manufacturer of Premarin was shocked and a lengthy reanalysis of the data was undertaken.

"Ten years later in 2011, the National Cancer Institute released data stating that with synthetic estrogen use (Premarin), the incidence of breast cancer was 23 percent lower than women taking a non-estrogen placebo. In addition, it was concluded that adding Provera definitely increased the incidences of breast cancer. Another study concluded a 69 percent increase in breast cancer when both Premarin and Provera were used. On the other hand, many studies have been done on bioidentical estrogen—on thousands of patients in fact—and the resulting data is excellent. It has been shown that natural progesterone actually prevents breast cancer and bioidentical estrogen either shows no increased risk of breast cancer or a slight decrease. In patients who have had breast cancer who use bioidentical hormones, numerous studies show survival is the same as patients using no hormones at all.

> *Carrying the Braca gene greatly increases the incidence of breast cancer, but this gene is responsible for only 5 to 10 percent of all breast cancer.*

Other studies show even better survival and fewer reoccurrences in patients using bioidentical hormones compared to non-hormone users. Let's look at some of the studies together."

I turn the pages of her notebook to "Causes of Breast Cancer" and we begin to review the studies together. I explain how low thyroid, high blood sugar, iodine deficiency, low D3, dairy consumption and being overweight all contribute significantly to increased breast cancer. Lauren has all of these risk factors.

The peak incidence of breast cancer occurs after a woman has had no estrogen exposure for approximately twenty-five years.

Cigarette smoking and other carcinogens such as mold, mercury and pest sprays also increase the risk for cancer in general, including breast cancer. Lauren has not exposed herself to these risk factors. Carrying the Braca gene greatly increases the incidence of breast cancer, but this gene is responsible for only 5 to 10 percent of all breast cancer. Where Lauren was tested because an aunt has breast cancer, she was found to be negative for the gene. I explain that if estrogen is involved in any increase in breast cancer it is because the liver sometimes breaks down the estrogen in unhealthy ways. We can detect that problem by monitoring estrogen breakdown with twenty-four-hour urine testing, then adding iodine and a supplement called EstroProtect if indicated.

I further explain that in patients not taking hormones the peak incidence of breast cancer is age seventy-four to seventy-nine. This means that the peak incidence of breast cancer occurs after a woman has had no estrogen exposure for approximately twenty-five years. Given the belief that estrogen causes breast cancer, why do young women, who have the highest estrogen levels, have such rare occurrences of breast cancer? We continue to discuss this complex topic and Lauren is fully engaged.

While we talk, I think back to my patients who have developed breast cancer while taking bioidentical hormones and am impressed that the number is so small. Few doctors prescribe as many bioidentical hormones as I do. I've prescribed them for thousands of patients for over thirty years. Given the incidence of one in seven women developing breast cancer in the Western world, literally hundreds and hundreds of my patients should have developed breast cancer. However, over thirty years of being in practice the number of women who have developed breast cancer among my patients is rare compared to the reported incidence of one out of seven women. Based on the size of a cancer, a radiologist can calculate how many years it has been growing, and I always discuss with the radiologist how long a patient's breast cancer has been present. Among my patients who have developed breast cancer while taking bioidentical hormones, the radiologists frequently indicate that cancer was present but too small to diagnose when they began taking the bioidentical hormones.

I have treated a large group of women like Lauren, who have had breast cancer and want hormonal treatment for their menopausal symptoms. In the practice of Western medicine prescribing

> *The number of women who have developed breast cancer among my patients is rare compared to the reported incidence of one out of seven women.*

hormones for these patients is generally discouraged. As studies accumulate on this subset of patients, I am grateful to tell my patients that many of them report that bioidentical estrogen does not increase reoccurrence rates. Some studies even show a decreased incidence of breast cancer reoccurrences compared to non-hormone users.

> *This advanced scanner takes more than 1800 ultrasound images per breast, and these images are then compressed into a movie. The accuracy is amazing, allowing the radiologist to see tiny cancers as small as several millimeters.*

Seven years ago I invited Dr. Kevin Kelley to practice at the Center. He is a brilliant breast radiologist who is creating a paradigm change in how to diagnose early breast cancer. During his illustrious career he was the head of breast imaging at Santa Monica hospital for years, and then a founder of the Hill Memorial Breast Center in Pasadena, where his group performed and read hundreds of mammograms each day. After years of dealing with the inaccuracies of mammography in women with dense breast tissue, and women's complaints about painful mammography, he created the groundbreaking SonoCine machine. This advanced scanner takes more than 1800 ultrasound images per breast and these images are then compressed into a movie. The accuracy is amazing, allowing the radiologist to see tiny cancers as small as several millimeters. The standard size that conventional mammography picks up is 7 to 15 mm. Having warm gel slathered like massage oil over the breasts causes no complaints either.

When Dr. Kelley arrived at the Center with his impressive machine, he went to work on our patients. At the end of a few months he came to me puzzled and worried. He hadn't diagnosed a single case of breast cancer and had been methodically ticking through what might have happened to the scanner during the move. The technicians had already come to check on the machine and found nothing wrong. I told him not to worry, because we rarely saw breast cancer at the Center—only one or two were diagnosed every few years. He was both astonished and puzzled. How could a Center prescribing so many hormones have so little breast cancer? This was his introduction to an understanding of bioidentical hormones, something still not understood by most doctors. A few months later he came to me beaming (and also apologizing for being so happy), because he was now diagnosing plenty of breast cancer, just like he did at his other locations. The cancer wasn't in our population of patients, but rather in patients who sought his care from the local community. He now has sixty machines in the United States and is clearly on the forefront of changing breast imaging from mammography to a SonoCine approach that exposes women to zero radiation. Everyday we image women using the SonoCine with confidence, knowing that if breast

> *The possibility must be considered that estrogen somehow protects breast tissue from developing cancer.*

> *"Estrogen builds muscle and rejuvenates skin, so we must ask ourselves whether the cellular health of breast tissue might also be enhanced by this hormone."*

cancer does arise it will be picked up in its earliest stages. Given Lauren's breast cancer history, I feel it is critical for her to be tested.

When examining the low breast cancer incidence in the Center, the possibility must be considered that estrogen somehow protects breast tissue from developing cancer. We know estrogen is a powerful inhibitor of osteoporosis. Within the first three years of menopause women lose large amounts of bone, paving the way for future osteoporosis and hip fractures. Muscles wasting and skin sagging are also standard findings after menopause. Estrogen builds muscle and rejuvenates skin, so we must ask ourselves whether the cellular health of breast tissue might also be enhanced by this hormone. In menopause, women also experience more insulin resistance and diabetes due to low estrogen. This causes cellular dysfunction and more cancer. Fifty percent of diabetic patients develop cancer. Bioidentical estrogen prevents 50 percent of diabetes in menopause, and therefore prevents many forms of cancer. Ninety percent of all cancer arises through or is aided by inflammation. What happens when a woman goes through menopause? Her inflammatory markers rise, along with arthritis, heart disease and dementia. All of these diseases have inflammation as one of their core causes. What happens to our adrenal glands in menopause? They become stressed and deficient, knocking out one of our body's primal defenses against cancer.

> *Ninety percent of all cancer arises through, or is aided by, inflammation. What happens when a woman goes through menopause? Her inflammatory markers rise, along with arthritis, heart disease and dementia.*

We need to help maintain our adrenal function and estrogen is an important contributor.

> *Estrogen is an amazing rejuvenator for women.*

By replacing menopausal patients' estrogen with bioidentical estrogens, these women experience decreased blood sugar, decreased stress and decreased inflammation. These are all great for cancer prevention, including breast cancer. Interestingly, elevations in a woman's stress, blood sugar and inflammation also increase the number one cause of death in women: heart attacks. Studies show that bioidentical estrogen prevents heart attack death in women. In my thirty years of prescribing bioidentical hormones only three patients have suffered a heart attack, and to date all three are doing well. And I am caring for older women with the highest risk of dying from breast cancer and heart attacks.

All of this means that estrogen is a critical hormone for preventing many of the diseases of aging in women. We need be open to its benefits and stop calling it the cancer-causing, disease-promoting bad guy. Estrogen is an amazing rejuvenator for women.

I share much of this information with Lauren and she now needs to make a decision. Should she try bioidentical hormones for her symptoms and disease prevention, or forego this treatment? Her decision will impact her life greatly.

"Lauren, we have discussed this in detail and you have read extensively. Do you want to ask your oncologists if they would agree to have you try a bit of estrogen cream? And really, if you don't want to, it's absolutely okay with me. I have alternative treatments that also work quite well in controlling symptoms."

Lauren shifts in her chair. "Prudence, it's such a hard choice, and it comes down to feeling reluctant right now. But I am so miserable! What other options do you have?"

"We can build your adrenal hormones, add thyroid, and give you some testosterone, all of which you are deficient in. And I don't think your oncologist would feel there's a controversy in terms of increasing breast cancer reoccurrence. For your menopausal symptoms. I have formulated a great set of Korean herbs called Feminine Radiance. Women in Korea report greatly reduced menopausal symptoms when they take these herb combinations. Lauren, there are so many natural, noncontroversial solutions to offer you. I don't believe women need to contract breast cancer, and they certainly don't need to die from it."

I feel bioidentical hormone use for patients with breast cancer is a reasonable and safe treatment plan for menopause.

"That's great news, Prudence, really heartening." Lauren's smile shows her relief. "I came here adamantly opposed to hormones, but I see the data has progressed well beyond my knowledge. Still, I'd like to take the least controversial approach. I'd like to start on all the other bioidentical hormones and I'd love to try Feminine Radiance. If I continue to feel this bad, I will probably try a small amount of bioidentical estrogen, because you're right that the studies look pretty neutral in terms of cancer reoccurrences. And I don't want to harm myself by not taking it. Boy, we are all in a bit of a bind, aren't we?"

I touch Lauren on the arm. "Each woman needs to evaluate her own situation and choose. I want to be clear that I feel bioidentical hormone use for patients with breast cancer is a reasonable and safe treatment plan for menopause. I also believe that we might be ten years ahead of the current standard of care for breast cancer. Standard-of-care protocols are not the gold standard by any means. They're frequently outdated and can be as much as twenty years behind the most effective treatments. But I respect the concerns raised about hormones and request that my breast cancer patients consult their oncologist, or perhaps get another opinion with one of the oncologists I recommend.

"In your case, Lauren, I have no doubt that you'll feel so much better with your other hormones balanced, even without estrogen. It is essential that you begin taking iodine, too. Iodine deficiency is a definite cause of breast cancer. Iodine-rich diet is one of the reasons Japanese women have so little breast cancer. Our iodine capsules have selenium in them too, which is also very helpful. And of course your thyroid is low which, when corrected, will also help prevent reoccurrences. One-half grain of Biothyroid is a good starting point. It contains both T3 and T4 and is a natural thyroid hormone. One Super Adrenal, which has three adrenal hormones as well as adrenal gland support, will help rebuild your adrenal glands."

I let Lauren know about our Path of Fulfillment workshops, which are offered in the evenings. She agrees that stress could have played a role in her breast cancer and is fascinated by the

WellBe watch that comes with her Immersion Program. She started wearing it during her day with us, and all day her stress level was 80-95 percent. It helps her interrupt the stress, which plummeted to below 35. She signs up for a meditation series with Anil Chandwani, and tells me her WellBe is acting much nicer to her—beeping only a few times a day. I know how important our emotions and thoughts are in staying well. In Lauren's case, her divorce ten years ago was extremely traumatic. She was married to a litigation attorney who ended up disowning her children and somehow wiggling out of all child or alimony support. Several homes she owned with her husband had been clandestinely sold and the common assets rendered untraceable. During that time she pieced together a web of deceit and sex addiction spanning more than ten years. What she believed was true love turned out to be true lies. Because of the extent of her trauma, I referred Lauren to Hazel Carter, a trauma specialist. I have seen her myself and she is an extremely gifted, dedicated practitioner.

Diet is critical for longevity and breast cancer prevention, so Lauren's next stop is with our naturopath who will individualize her diet toward cancer prevention. I am sure our patients have so few occurrences of breast cancer because we use an integrated approach, correcting and adjusting every aspect of health related to cancer.

Dr. Nikki, one of our Naturopathic physicians, takes Lauren off the dairy products, she heavily relied upon as her protein source, and encourages her to be grain- and gluten-free. Her hemoglobin A1C is 5.8, which indicates she is insulin resistant and bordering on being diabetic. It also is a cause of increased breast cancer. She is given a kit to test her stool for parasites, candida and other problems. Both poor health and dreaded diseases like cancer arise from faulty intestinal health.

At the end of these consults, our educator meets with Lauren to make sure she understands the program and when to return for her second appointment.

As Lauren leaves, I see her at the front desk looking much happier. She gives me a hug, her eyes filling with tears. "Thank you, Prudence. I have new hope and I think I'll be able to do all this. It's not that hard, and then I will get healthy and become beautiful again." She gives me a hopeful smile, this time without cynicism or doubt.

Two weeks later, Lauren calls with the following feedback: her fatigue is lifting a bit, the hot flashes have diminished, and she is not so depressed. She has no bad reactions to the supplements. Everything is good, and we will see how she feels at one month.

When I see Lauren's name on the schedule a month later, I am eager to catch up and further her plan. "Hello, Lauren!" I beam. "How's life going for you?"

> *"The weight will start to come off once we help you heal your digestive system."*

She greets me like a long-lost relative. "Prudence! I am better. I only have a few hot flashes every day, not twenty like I used to, and I'm sleeping better. I also have more energy. I still don't feel like I used to when I was younger, but really, any amount of improvement is good."

We sit together and I continue. "That's great! I am so happy you feel better. The good news is that we can make you feel even better because your recent blood work still shows deficiencies." I open her notebook and add the new page that shows her current values. "See how your thyroid is better, but not ideal? Let's add another half grain and see how you feel. Your adrenals are better but still low. Begin two Super Adrenals. Your D3 is still disastrously low, although it is improving. Low D3 increases the risk of breast cancer, so please begin taking two D3 pills. Is that all okay?"

"Easy," she replies, then drops her head. "But I haven't lost weight yet!"

"You will once your body begins to rebuild from your difficult menopause. You are scheduled to see Dr. Nikki again today, and she will go over your stool test. You actually have a parasite and H. Pylori, which make weight loss harder. The weight will start to come off once we help you heal your digestive system. We need to be vigilant with your breast health, and that means losing weight and lowering your sugar levels. Have you had your SonoCine yet?"

Lauren looks sheepish and confesses she hasn't had time. "Why not now?" I ask her, and she happily agrees. "But I did make an appointment with Hazel and adore her. I've had three sessions. She is so busy I'm lucky to have gotten in. I see how my divorce was a repetition of an older abuse pattern, and I am moving through this. We are doing EMDR and Brain Spotting. Really,

I am grateful to her. Oh, and I am coming to Anil's meditation evenings. I like meditating!"

"Wonderful, just wonderful. Why don't you check out Mentors Channel and expand your meditation a bit. They have some of the most wonderful teachers offering programs all month long. I'm always involved with them. Right now, I just finished the OSHO program which was free for twenty-one days, and I bought more lectures. I listen while I am driving or doing my yoga. Truly, Doron Libshtein, who founded Mentors Channel, and that whole group is amazing." I write down mentorschannel. com in her book. After more talk, she goes in to see Petra to figure out why she hasn't lost weight yet.

The next day I get a call from Dr. Kelly who has read the SonoCine scan we did yesterday. "Prudence, it's not good news. Lauren has what looks like a small reoccurrence. At 5 mm, it has been there for more than two years. The good news is that all the lymph nodes look good, so she will only need a small excision of the tumor and most likely nothing else. When we pick these things up under one centimeter, chemo and radiation are almost never needed." I make the difficult call to Lauren and explain what Dr. Kelly has told me.

"Oh my God," Lauren's voice is shaking, "I can't believe this!"

"I'm so sorry, Lauren. This really is scary but it is completely curable, and there will only be a tiny scar. It is sad that you are revisiting this trauma. How is WellBe acting?"

I sense Lauren smile over the phone. "Well, Mr. WellBe is not happy. He is telling me right now in fact, that I need to start breathing. My stress is at 89 percent."

I do a little breathing with Lauren, and her stress falls.

"So Lauren, we need to find out why cancer is forming in your breast and we need to have this little one removed. Do you want to see your same surgeon? Do you want to see the doctor who did your last surgery?"

Lauren responds with a weak yes, and after more encouragement and support says she will make an appointment the next day. My staff calls her back the following day and she confirms she has an appointment with the oncologist in a week. She is not feeling as frantic.

I see Lauren a week later and give her a big hug. "Your surgeon called and said it was a tiny little cancer. Now it is gone completely. How are you doing with all this?"

Lauren pauses and then looks me right in the eyes. "Not so good. It is exactly what Dr. Kelly said. Just 4 mm but I'm very, very scared."

"I understand. It is frightening to be faced with this again. But the good news is that if a breast cancer is detected under one centimeter, a woman has the same survival as a woman without cancer. And she doesn't need chemo or radiation. Cancer doubles in size each year, so Dr. Kelly said it's been growing for more than two years. I am so happy it was picked up so early due to the

SonoCine's accuracy. How do you feel about the recommendation of having a double mastectomy?"

Lauren exhales a deep breath and hangs her head. "Well, my surgeon is recommending that because it seems like they also found some other areas of pre-cancer; they called it DCIS. They said I'm cancer-prone and shouldn't take any further risks." She then looks at me and I can see determination in her eyes. "I'm not happy at all about that recommendation. I'm not going to do it. I don't want to lose my breasts. Dr. Kelly said it was so small he could treat it with only a tiny excision. Mastectomies would be a nightmare, a real triple whammy. I would be a breast-less, menopausal, double cancer survivor."

"Oh Lauren, that really doesn't sound like a good scenario. It sounds so traumatic. Have you told Hazel yet?"

"Yeah, I went yesterday, and I always feel so much better after seeing her. Today I am positively cheery compared to yesterday. This pattern of loss is *going* to stop. She is taking me back to very early trauma where all this probably started."

I smile with reassurance. "Good, Lauren, good. We are all on a journey, and the question to ask is why you are at this juncture. Why are you here? What do you need to see?"

"I have been in that inquiry. I keep asking myself why." Lauren sits up straight.

"Any answers yet?" I tilt my head.

"I have lots of ideas, but they are still kind of vague and swirling around in my head. I'm going to work on that in my meditations."

"Great idea. Answers come in that stillness, as well as from your guides and trusted source. Once you know why you arrived again at this cancer juncture, you won't need to return to this place any more. Did your doctor give you any ideas about why this reoccurred?"

Lauren shakes her head. "She had no idea. I did everything they told me to do the first time and took all the chemo and radiation. She said the incidence of breast cancer is rising that we just don't know why so many women are getting it. It was a very unsatisfying answer."

She pauses for a few moments. "But I think I know why it came back. I have been doing too much work not to know. I didn't change my lifestyle. I continued to eat sugar and dairy. I am overweight. And I really shouldn't have gone through menopause for these last four or five years without hormones. My body got all out of whack. That's why everything was so off when I came to see you the first time. I have been reading non-stop since I first saw you, but I just didn't understand what happens to a woman in menopause. One of my friends is a PhD and she did a literature search for me. You're right. Literally hundreds of studies have been done about women taking bioidentical hormones, and it's not a bad choice. In fact, I've decided to take some estrogen … is that okay?"

> *"Well, estradiol is great for your brain. You'll see your brilliant brain come back."*

"Of course. I respect your decision and feel it's a valid one." I reach for a pad of paper from my desk. "I'll give you the names of a few oncologists who have an open mind about this issue."

Lauren sits back in her chair. "Good, because my oncologist has been very clear that she won't let me try any estrogen. But the thing is I am going to do it because it no longer works for me to have a doctor 'let me do something.' This is not how I talk to my employees and this is not how I talk to my friends. This attitude is outdated. I also believe estrogen will help decrease risk of cancer and also help counteract the damage the chemo did to me. I feel like I'm losing my brain function. I have what women call 'chemo-brain,' and I am probably getting dementia from it."

> *PuraZymes are the best enzymes I know. They help heal the digestive tract and get rid of any plaque you may have in your intestines. Plaque is a breeding ground for cancer.*

"Well, estradiol is great for your brain," I reply. "You'll see your brilliant brain come back. In fact, let's put you on the supplement I formulated called Brilliant Brain. It will help your brain recover faster."

A few weeks later I receive a letter from Lauren's new oncologist who agrees to have her use a small amount of bioidentical estrogen cream. He would feel much better if Lauren agreed to do a double mastectomy, but he will support her decision. I send Lauren her low dose bioidentical estrogen from our dispensary, and one month later she arrives at the Center to see me. She feels much more energetic, the depression is lifting, and she is finally sleeping. We sit in chairs close to each other and she shares her latest news.

"Prudence, I can't believe how much better I feel. I was so bad back when I first saw you that I didn't even realize how horrible I was feeling. And my brain is a little better. It's quite amazing."

We celebrate these small victories and then I tell her we really need to get serious about cancer prevention. We need to add systemic enzymes and coffee enemas to her regimen. "Lauren, PuraZymes are systemic enzymes that need to be taken on an empty stomach. They eat up any inflammation and cancer cells that may be present. We all have cancer cells in our bodies, but they just never make it to the stage where they cause problems. PuraZymes are the best enzymes I know. They have an important place in all cancer therapy. They help heal the digestive tract and get rid of any plaque you may have in your intestines. Plaque is a breeding ground for cancer."

Lauren says she is faithfully taking her digestive enzymes and will take the systemic enzymes too. Next, we discuss finding her a doctor who specializes in cancer. "Lauren, I'm not a cancer doctor. I help prevent cancer and reoccurrences, but there are some great doctors who specialize in this field. Have you seen Suzanne Somers's book called *Knock Out?* It is a wonderful resource."

"I saw it in your store, but didn't know it was about cancer. I'll take any help I can get."

"I like Dr. James Forsythe in Reno." I smile as quick memories of Dr. Forysthe flash through my mind. "He has an integrated approach to cancer as well as a great track record. I'm so sorry I can't refer you to Dr. Gonzalez. He recently died, and was an incredible cancer doctor. His passing is a loss to the world. About the mastectomy recommendation, I don't want you to do anything you're not ready for. On the one hand, studies have shown that DCIS is fairly common and usually doesn't progress to breast cancer. One study done in England, for example, found DCIS in 40 percent of women under the age of forty. Treating them all with mastectomies would result in a lot of missing breasts.

"On the other hand, for some women it is the right choice. However, regardless of what choice is made, a mastectomy is not a comprehensive way to treat this disease process. It is a little like painting the leaves on a sick tree green, rather than watering and fertilizing the roots. It is essential to

> *A mastectomy is not a comprehensive way to treat this disease process. It is a little like painting the leaves on a sick tree green, rather than watering and fertilizing the roots.*

change your cellular health from the inside. Digestive enzymes, systemic enzymes, IV nutrients, coffee enemas, D3, restoring immunity, gut restoration and detox all create cellular health. We need to continue working on your digestion and can build on what you're doing with your diet. Dr. Petra will keep working with you. Digestive health is critical for good health and cancer prevention."

I watch Lauren's brow furrow. "Prudence, this sounds more and more complicated. I hope I can do it all."

"I understand. This new diagnosis really ups the ante, and I agree this comprehensive cleanup-and-rebalance phase is complex. But you're past the hard part. Maintenance is easy. It's a process. Little by little this all becomes routine. And you will lose the excess weight and grow more beautiful, super healthy and happy."

"Okay, I'm in." Lauren's confidence returns. "Just tell me what to do so I don't mess up and forget things. My brain is better but still not that smart yet."

I walk Lauren out of the office and our naturopath takes over. She will work with Lauren for several months to make sure she is losing weight and healing her digestion. After that appointment, our patient educator sits with Lauren and goes over her hormonal and gut restoration programs to make sure she understands what needs to be done. The regimen is clear and concise.

In our practitioner meetings, our Naturopathic doctor, Dr. Nikki, tells me Lauren's gas and bloating are gone, and that she is being incredible with her diet. She cheats once in a while, but loves the avocados, good oils, fruits, and tons of veggies her diet includes.

I see Lauren two months later and she looks shiny and happy. She also feels stronger. She is exercising and has lost fourteen pounds, making a huge difference in her appearance.

"Lauren, I have been following you these last months through Hazel and Dr. Nikki and am so impressed! Tell me all about yourself."

She smiles and reaches out to me with energy. "Well, I'm happier. No more menopause and the weight is coming off. I feel patient with the kids and balanced. It's like a tsunami hit my body three months ago and now the damage has been cleared away. Really, I feel better, and my brain is starting to work much better."

I take her hand in mine. "That's just great! You look amazing and I am so proud of you. It's been a lot of hard work and you've stuck with all the changes amazingly well."

Lauren giggles. "It wasn't hard. When you get a diagnosis like cancer, you suddenly realize how precious life is. But the thing is, before doing this work, I didn't feel life was so precious. In a very subconscious way, I might have even been hoping to leave. Prudence, I didn't realize how much trauma I had experienced. I was raised to ignore my emotions and sadness. Boy, not anymore! And as I feel more, I am coming alive, and I want to live a very, very long time!"

"Good. I want you to as well," I chime in. "Maybe you'll come hiking in the Himalayas with me and Suzanne Somers when we're 120. We need an attorney on our team."

Lauren throws her head back and laughs. "Great, I'm in. I'll make sure the team members sign a liability release. I can be very useful. But how do my hormones look—my lab values?"

I open her notebook and turn it so she can see. "Almost perfect. Really shipshape. Your D3 is now seventy-two, which is great; your FSH is down to thirteen; and the estrogen level is super. Your twenty-four hour urine test says you're breaking down your estrogen correctly, which helps prevent breast cancer. And your adrenals are healing too. They're still a little off, so let's raise your dose to one Mega Adrenal each morning, which equals three Super Adrenals. And be sure to stay on your iodine protocol for three months and your Estro Protect supplement. Estro Protect helps you break your estrogen down safely. Let's continue testing your thyroid every few months with the Thyroflex. That iodine protocol is an amazing and simple way to prevent breast cancer reoccurrences, but we might need to adjust your thyroid dose from time to time. Are you still feeling tired at all?"

Lauren shakes her head. "Nope. I've actually cut back my hours at work. This corporation stuff is not chicken soup for the soul. I was probably trying to please my father or something when I went to law school. I need a new direction—new work that is meaningful."

I sit in silence for a few moments thinking about her first words to me: "I just can't believe this is all there is." I remember thinking, *Oh, boy ... she is calling in a new life; this is going to be the real reason she came here.*

> *"Living your life's purpose and experiencing everything you need to experience is why you came here."*

"Of course, Lauren! Living your life's purpose and experiencing everything you need to experience is why you came here. How are you doing with that?"

She sits back for a few seconds. "Well, I'm meditating, and I love Mentors Channel. I buy their programs and have gone through several of them a number of times. I'm changing, or I guess *growing* is the right word. I took Tim Kelley's 'True Purpose' interactive program on the site. I have this feeling I need to work with him."

"I know Tim and he is wonderful. He is one of the mentors working with Doron Libshtein. Yes, he is direct, clear and inspiring. If you want, I'll ask Doron if Tim is taking on new clients."

Lauren lights up and beams like a smiling Buddha. We hug and say goodbye, and I jot myself a note to talk with Doron. Later, he tells me Tim is taking on new clients—usually people involved in global transformation—and if it's a good fit, he'll take a new client. If it's not a good fit he has other mentors to suggest.

⌒

The stream of life moves rapidly, and six months pass before I see Lauren again. I look at her with astonishment. She is beautiful—tall and willowy. "Wow, Lauren wow! What happened to you? How are you?"

"Life happened, Prudence." We sit together and she takes my hand. "Life grabbed me, shook me and claimed me. I am not the same person any more. I've been working with Tim Kelley and have made a career change. I realized I'm actually happiest being in a more social 'people' field. I also like to create and call the shots in my life."

"I loathed the corporate world. I find it so interesting how rapidly change can happen. I'm happy to announce I'm now creating a foundation to help teenage orphans in Nepal. I love to travel, and I love children. On a trip to Nepal years ago, I felt heartbroken by the homeless kids. I looked into it and the orphanages can only keep them until they are fifteen, after which then the kids have to leave and work. But the thing is they don't have skills. So I'm starting a halfway house for fifteen-to twenty-one-year-olds.

Lauren smiles like she has a secret to share. "You mentioned the Shanti Houses in Israel and I looked them up. I have talked quite a bit with Mariuma, and now I am going to do something similar.

I have spent three months in Nepal already, and we're taking over an old factory and making it into the home. There is so much to do and I'm busy nonstop, but it is a different kind of busyness than before. This is so much fun. This is who I am! It is a Nepalese project and there are so many good people involved. It will be a combined project with East meeting West. Volunteers will come to Nepal to teach life and work skills, then we'll export their crafts and ideas to the West. It will create business opportunities. Also, my kids love Nepal. It feels good to get them out of San Francisco."

She reaches into her bag, takes out a small wrapped gift and hands it to me beaming. "You really are making a difference in the world. Not just with me, but with so many people. Thank you. I can't express how full my heart feels. I am so grateful."

I remove the little ribbons and out billows a soft, pale pink, lovely cashmere scarf like a delicate cloud of beauty. My eyes fill with tears as I put it on. "Lauren, it is just gorgeous ... beautiful! You are a gift to me. I will treasure this. Thank you."

We go over all her lab values and I make a few minor adjustments in her thyroid hormones. Her pelvic ultrasound is normal, and she is hiking, eating well and hopefully not picking up new parasites in Nepal. We will do a spot check stool test to make sure. She has seen her oncologist faithfully and has done another SonoCine with Dr. Kelly and it looks great. Things look very positive. Her oncologist is no longer telling her she needs mastectomies. We finish our consult and part for another six months.

Five years pass and Lauren continues to thrive. There is no return of her cancer and she feels strong, smart and healthy. She spends half her time in Nepal, and she has married an Irish doctor who has been in Nepal for years attending to both rich and poor alike. She arrives at this consult with another small gift. It is a weaving from their Nepalese workshop and it is offered in celebration of being breast cancer free for five years. It is a powerful milestone to pass and we celebrate by meeting at Gratitude Café after work. We discuss our work and the friendship we have developed. I want to hear all about her newest project.

I think back over the nine years I have known Lauren. She remains cancer free, with perfect mammograms and normal SonoCines. Lauren tells me cancer is a thing of the past and I believe her. She has done the deep inner work and made the necessary physical changes to heal. She is in love, and loving and living her life's true purpose while doing all the necessary things to remain physically healthy. Her stress is very low and her diet is excellent. She has maintained her meditation practices and her exercise is neither too strenuous nor too sporadic. In short, she approached this cancer problem by integrating the physical, emotional and spiritual aspects of herself, and made the changes needed to save her life. In turn, she is saving the lives of her Nepalese orphans. One life saved in order to save many lives.

I think back to the many patients with breast cancer whom I have helped with menopause over the years. My job is to let women know their options, offer resources and help guide them to their greatest possible health. Like Lauren initially did, some women elect to balance all their hormones except estrogen. Others beg for estrogen and tell me even if they die earlier because of it, at least they will have some good years. I tell them they don't have to die from feeling good, and the hormonal balance causing them to feel good can also boost their immunity, decrease inflammation and, in many cases, decrease reoccurrences. This is backed by hundreds of studies as well as by my experience with patients. One of my missions in life is to help as many women as I can be vital, healthy, beautiful and sensual their whole lives, and women with breast cancer must not be left behind.

Takeaway for breast cancer and menopause:

Breast cancer arises from many sources including low D3, low iodine intake, low production of thyroid hormones and a diet high in dairy, gluten, sugar and soy. Stress is strongly implicated in breast cancer, which means we need to monitor and decrease our stress. Most traditional oncologists believe estrogen causes breast cancer and follow a strategy to eliminate all of a woman's natural estrogen with drugs. If estrogen can be implicated in breast cancer, it is most likely due to an improper detoxification of estrogen, which can be corrected. Monitoring estrogen metabolites with 24-hour urine (Meridian Valley is excellent) easily identifies any unhealthy metabolites. DIM (broccoli extract), Calcium D Glucarate, and iodine all help push estrogen towards healthy metabolites. Eliminating estrogen from a woman's body results in more inflammation, more internal stress, and higher blood sugar levels, which are all independent causes of cancer in general. This cut and burn strategy oncologists take with eliminating estrogen throws the baby out with the bathwater and places a woman at significant risk for heart attacks (the number one cause of death in women) and dementia. New research has implicated the human papillary virus (HPV) in breast cancer. Maintaining a healthy immunity is critical to keep this and other viruses at bay. Our digestive tract is a breeding ground for inflammation. Parasites, yeast, *leaky gut*, and H. Pylori all need to be identified and corrected. Heavy metals are implicated in many cancers and breast cancer is no exception. It is not difficult to identify and gently detoxify industrial toxicity from our bodies.

Prescription for breast cancer and menopause:

- Balance all hormones back to healthy levels with bioidentical natural hormones.

- Create a talented, supportive team of doctors and practitioners around you.

- Begin an impeccable, anti-inflammatory, anti-angiogenesis diet.

- Lose any excess weight and begin a healthy exercise routine.

- Heal and restore the gut to excellent health.

- Screen for heavy metals toxicity and detox gently and naturally if required.

- Do IV nutrient and cancer preventing supplementation, such as the iodine protocol.

- Do the inner deep work needed to resolve past trauma and emotional issues.

- Receive and give love in all ways possible.

- Live your life's true purpose in alignment with who you are.

- Wear the WellBe stress bracelet to monitor and treat stress.

- Meditate.

- Do yoga and spiritual practices to keep you centered and joyful.

- Begin the iodine protocol if you have recently been diagnosed with breast cancer.

- Begin taking Biodine to help prevent breast cancer.

- Estro-Protect: 2 capsules per day

- D3: 5000-10,000 IU per day

- Inflam Alleve: 2-4 capsules per day to reduce inflammation

- PuraZymes: 4-5 capsules on an empty stomach, 3 times per day

Chapter 9

Divine Eros

Elizabeth arrives early with her husband, and they sit on my couch talking while I finish up with my prior patient. When I see couples, I know relationship issues will surely come up, and I feel an uneasy energy between them as I sit down. Did one of them drag the other to this consult? Have they been fighting? Has one of them had an affair?

"Hello, I'm Prudence. It's so nice to meet you Elizabeth, and David, right?"

We shake hands and I pull up my chair, ready to listen. "Thanks for coming in to see me. I hope you didn't wait too long."

Elizabeth jumps in. "We were early, and I'm so glad you could see us. I've been having problems for a number of years now, and David agreed to come with me. He's so busy at work, but this is important to us. We've been married twenty-two years, and I'm just not feeling like myself."

"I'm so sorry, Elizabeth. Let's see what we can do to bring you back."

Elizabeth leans in. "Well, I'm forty-five, and we have two kids, fifteen and seventeen years old. I spend long hours as a television producer and David is in feature films, so I guess you'd say our schedules are insane. I have good energy. I'm not depressed and I sleep well, so I don't think I'm in perimenopause. But the thing is … I just don't have any interest in sex. It's becoming a big issue because, well, David is only forty-three, and he wants to make love all the time. I mean, every day! I shouldn't be saying this with David in the room, but I fake it all the time. I love him, and I used to feel really sexy and ready, but I now have no sex drive at all … actually, not for the last three years."

I lean in to meet her body language. "I'm so sorry, Elizabeth. I understand." I glance at David and offer him a brief, reassuring smile. "Each day women express to me their distress over this kind of thing. You are not alone and there are many medical causes for a low libido. I know you're not happy being in a conflict with your honey over something so important. You've actually done really well. Twenty-two years of marriage is a long time! Did anything seem to cause this dwindling desire?"

"Well, with kids and work, things go by fast. And I've been busy, so I don't think any one thing really started the problem. Maybe I was more tired a few years ago because I was on a challenging series, but now things are more even keeled. I just don't seem to have great orgasms either. It's hard for me to want to make love in the first place, but then when I finally do, it's not so great. I hope something is wrong that can be corrected."

"We'll look at everything, Elizabeth." I touch her arm. "It is a complex topic, but to start with, how much are you actually making love these days?"

"Well, it feels like a lot," Elizabeth volunteers. "I guess about once a week and Prudence, he's such a good guy. He doesn't pressure me."

I hear a sigh from David. He looks at Elizabeth with his face scrunched up. "Really, it's never, I mean, once every two or three weeks at the most. We have very little time together. In the past, when we found time, we'd fall into each other's arms and make love, even at the expense of

> "Whole countries have been lost over a woman's Yoni."

other things. It was quick and we both felt happy and renewed. Making love is like a mini-vacation. I guess the more pressure I'm under the more I need to make love."

David sits back in his chair. "Elizabeth seems to be the opposite. She now prefers we talk and I stroke her arm, and that's all. That's okay, it's just that she's really shut down. I keep trying new things to help her along but I guess I'm out of ideas."

I glanced between the two of them, sensing the uneasy energy. "So, it's too much sex for Elizabeth and not nearly enough for David. Sounds about right for the difference between masculine and feminine desire. So, what have you tried?"

"Well," David says, "I got some toys, like a vibrator, and I got some sexy videos. We've gone away for the night to get away from the kids … but it's kind of dead."

Elizabeth jumps in. "Yes, dead! He's right. I just would rather eat in bed than make love."

"Elizabeth, my dear, this is a troubling problem. Whole countries have been lost over a woman's Yoni."

"Yoni?" they both exclaim at once.

I smile. "Oh, sorry, it's becoming such a common word these days. 'Yoni' is a Sanskrit word for a woman's vagina. It denotes the creative power of nature moving the energy of the entire universe. It represents the goddess Shakti and is the origin of life, fertility, a woman's womb with all its life force."

> *The sacred union of the masculine and feminine energies are respected and worshipped in many temples in India because life is sacred, and new life arising out of that union is sacred. It goes well beyond sexual union.*

They ponder what I have said. Elizabeth is the first to speak. "Oh, I don't know much about Hinduism, but we were in India for a production shoot and saw some Lingim Yonis, or was it Shiva Lingims? The image of the masculine and feminine united sexually is, well, a bit bizarre."

I consider Elizabeth's word and remember when I used to ponder these images and be quite taken with them. The sacred union of the masculine and feminine energies is respected and worshipped in many temples in India because life is sacred, and new life arising out of that union is sacred. It goes well beyond sexual union. The deepest love arising from united masculine-feminine energy is what is worshipped, because it allows the universe to function as it is meant to do. I understand this union, and I want Elizabeth and David to feel that ancient truth.

I muse out loud. "I love that the Hindu God Shiva sat alone in meditation for thousands of years before Parvati felt his energy and joined him—not as a lesser God, but as the source of his energy. She is the divine feminine. Elizabeth, this is your correct alignment with David, as his energy. The problem you present today is not just about a mismatch of sexual energies, but rather about you flowering into the powerful presence of who you are. As that, lovemaking is the creative, regenerating force of the world. Did you feel any of that Life Force in India when you were there?"

They look at each other. "Well … yes. There is movement and energy in the land. It feels ancient, and the temples are truly alive with worshippers and fragrance. We felt the energy of centuries of devotion, unlike churches here."

"Yes, I agree. There is a Life Force in India that is palpable. It is also in Israel, by the way—two ancient countries. We have that Life Force, that primal kundalini energy as it is called, within each of us. The Hindus access it through their devotional practices, yoga, rituals and ceremonies; it is an integral part of their life. When a person's kundalini energy is completely awakened from the root chakra to the crown chakra, certain cultures consider that person 'enlightened.' This Life Force energy is a sexual energy, but more importantly, it is the connecting energy of Oneness. But the western world turned away from this big picture of 'all life as sexual energy.'

"Like in The Matrix, we chose the blue pill. Do you remember when Morpheus said, 'You take the blue pill—the story ends, you wake up in your bed and believe whatever you want to believe.'"

They both laugh and I feel our energy lightening.

"Here in the West, we are guided by the movie industry that is pumping out blue pill stuff, touting youth, external beauty, and 'sexiness,'" I tease. "But really, ecstatic union is the expression of

> *All realities are important: the physical, emotional and spiritual.*

and bridge back to our true nature. I want you to experience this in your lovemaking. On an energetic level we are all God, divine ecstasy, and radiance. So to view your sexual challenge only from a mechanical viewpoint would be a great error. Are you tracking with me?"

Elizabeth speaks up. "Yes. At times I have felt energy within me. When I was pregnant, for example, I experienced the world's creative energy alive within me. I guess I haven't concentrated my energies on it in a long time, and maybe that lack of attention and understanding has taken me away from being an expression of this expanded love you describe."

"Excellent, Elizabeth." I flash her a wide smile. "When we give our attention to something, it builds and becomes stronger. I want you both to think and dream about sex, and for sure I'll give you some practices to enhance it."

Elizabeth and David nod their heads with new energy. They get it. This understanding can shift their lovemaking to create a deeper, more ecstatic union.

"Okay, let's now approach this from a practical level and make sure all your hormones are working and the mechanical causes of poor orgasms are addressed. I've come to understand that in order to have the highest and best outcome all aspects are equally important: the physical, emotional and spiritual.

"On the physical level, let's look at your blood tests." I open their new patient workbook and turn it so they can see each page. "You can see exactly where you should be. I see three hormonal causes for your low libido, Elizabeth. Your testosterone is low, your thyroid is a tad off and so is your DHEA. Testosterone and DHEA are androgens (male hormones) that drive the female sexual response. I could also make the point that you are in the early stages of perimenopause, and that your slightly low estrogen value is also responsible for your low libido. Do you know about the work I do here with hormones in terms of adjusting them back to ideal levels?"

"Oh, yes, that's why we're here. I know all about bioidentical hormones, and I also know Suzanne Somers. She is just wonderful!"

I smile, reflecting on my good friend. "Yes! She is a good guru and my dear colleague. Thanks, Elizabeth, for being up to speed on this topic. I love educated patients. So, let's create a plan where I prescribe testosterone cream, a half grain of natural thyroid, iodine, and my Super Adrenal, which not only has DHEA but also pregnenolone and herbs to enhance your libido and overall energy. And I forgot to ask, do you get PMS?"

"Tons!" Elisabeth responds. "It started a few years ago and I turn into a real b-i-t-c-h a week before my period. I cry and get depressed, am super irritable, bloated, and I'm tired and sleep really poorly."

David cringes, and Elizabeth clenches her hands.

"Not good for sex, is it? Well, rather than being that 'B' word, I'd rather you become Kali. Look it up; it's much more powerful! But really, Elizabeth, this kind of PMS hallmarks the beginning of perimenopause and a woman's libido takes a huge dive in perimenopause and menopause. Women enter perimenopause in their late thirties and early forties, and you're right at that age. Actually, you're doing very well with this. I have helped literally thousands of menopausal and perimenopausal women get their libidos back, and I consider it a very important part of my work. To correct your estrogen deficiency let's give you small amounts of estrogen cream to apply the week before your period. It should get rid of that PMS hurdle. My RN will explain how to use these natural hormones. Does this sound like something you can do?"

"Yes," Elizabeth shakes her head vigorously, looking like she has some hope back.

> "I have helped literally thousands of menopausal and perimenopausal women get their libidos back, and I consider it a very important part of my work."

"Good. The next part is important too, because it is about the mechanics of orgasms and libido. You had vaginal births, right?" Elizabeth nods. "After a woman has a baby she needs to do Kegel exercises to get her yoni back in shape. If you didn't do those exercises, it's likely your vagina has lost muscle tone—and those same muscles are responsible for healthy, strong orgasms. Orgasms are simply the sensation of the pelvic floor muscles contracting."

"I tried Kegels but couldn't really get the muscles to contract." Elizabeth glances at the floor. "And yes, I feel my muscle tone is not like it used to be."

"Let's get those muscles in shape," I encourage. "I want you to put half your dose of testosterone right across your clitoris, at the base of your vagina, between the vaginal opening and your rectum." I show her a diagram so she's clear on the exact location. "And then I want you to get the exercise machine I have in the store to give your vaginal muscles a workout. The machine emits a light electrical current that causes your muscles to contract. When you feel them contract, I want you to contract even harder using your own force. This is really effective in building muscle tone. Do this five nights a week for fifteen minutes each night and in a few weeks you'll feel your muscular gripping power return. Weak vaginal muscles cause weak orgasms. Many of my patients couldn't have an orgasm at all before using testosterone and the Kegel machine. Are you ready to try this?"

"Sure. I'll give anything a try. I was actually thinking about having surgery for vaginal reconstruction. One of my friends said it really made a huge difference in her ability to orgasm."

"In my former life as a gynecological surgeon, I regularly performed surgery. It can be quite effective. It's called a posterior repair, and in the hands of a good surgeon, women who have been really torn and stretched by having babies can be helped. But first try your Kegel exercises with your machine. It's not invasive like surgery and does wonders for orgasms. I want you to feel virtuous if you have an orgasm while exercising your muscles. Orgasms exercise those muscles really effectively, so the more orgasms you have the stronger the muscle tone will be."

"Oh, goodie!" Elizabeth smiles and glances at David.

David and I both look at her. I haven't heard "oh, goodie" in a long time, and we all break into laughter.

"Okay, Team O, let's add more orgasmic power. I'm going to prescribe a cream called Dream Cream. After your shower at night, dry off and massage a dose into your clitoris; it's an amino acid mixture that dilates your blood vessels in your labial area, causing your orgasms to be stronger and more rapid. Also, I also want to prescribe oxytocin lozenges, Which are potent orgasm stimulators. Oxytocin is the safe 'love' hormone I have been prescribing to my patients for years. It's released naturally during sexual play and penetration, causing faster arousal … and orgasms. If you don't feel aroused, you'll never begin to make love in order to get the natural release of oxytocin, so taking a bit of

> *Oxytocin is the safe 'love' hormone I have been prescribing to my patients for years. It's released naturally during sexual play and penetration, causing faster arousal … and orgasms.*

oxytocin in the evening will get you into the mood before getting into bed."

I look over at David who is fully engaged in the conversation. "David, when you make love, start by rubbing Elizabeth's whole body and then gently twist and stimulate her nipples—not just for a minute, but maybe for five or ten minutes. She will not be able to resist you with all that oxytocin nipple stimulation releases. It also results in quicker and stronger orgasms. Want to give all that a try?"

David faces Elizabeth. "Honey, I am your nipple man. I will deliver you from this bondage and perdition of punkie orgasms." He extends his arm like a knight to a damsel in distress.

"Great David," I deadpan, "I'm sure you are more than equipped for this mission." David nods in a serious and manly way, and our beautiful Elizabeth graciously bows her head. They are game, and I think about how beautiful this will be for them as a couple.

"Okay, dear lovers, that's a lot of training for right now, and to keep learning at home I encourage you to buy a few books: *Love, Sex and Intimacy* by Mark Whitwell is great, and the tantric books in the store for women and men are also good. There is homework involved in this endeavor! And by the way, Dawn Cartright's immersion workshop is coming up. She is a lovely tantric teacher and this workshop focuses on women's practices. If you're free, Elizabeth, she's going to dive deep with all of us."

Elizabeth and David smile, and we all hug. While this was a lot of information, it is a necessary foundation for what is to come.

As they leave, I think about a patient I saw earlier today who, like Elizabeth, had been beaten down by years of hard work. Genevive started as a top executive in an investment company and traveled the world as a businesswoman. When she came to me for the first time she was single, depressed and exhausted by her thousands of miles of traveling, and really beginning to show her age. She had taken up drinking wine every evening and confessed she was getting worried about her isolation and what she perceived as becoming invisible to men. Genevive despaired that at fifty-eight she was done with life. She had been so driven by work and she had completely ignored herself.

We began by taking Genevive out of menopause with bioidentical hormones. Next, we set her up on a great diet, then had her meet with Doron Libshtein of Mentors Channel. Together they discussed who she truly was and her life's purpose, not who she was conditioned to be. She became so excited by dreams she had long ago forgotten that she retired from her demanding job and began a new life. Genevive started a foundation to help single women become entrepreneurs, began tango dancing and grew her hair down her shoulders. She also started going to transformational workshops and would tell me she didn't know where all the tears came from. After signing up online men started asking her out, and it was her policy to accept most dates as practice sessions. In the beginning, she would talk to her dates as

> *She stopped giving men advice and became an avid listener. Lo and behold, men began clamoring for her attention.*

she had always done with her male colleagues—competing with them, joking, and elaborating on their stories with her own successes. After analyzing those dates and realizing those men weren't asking her out again, Genevive took a few women's workshops with Michaela Boehm and became vulnerable and beautifully feminine. She stopped giving men advice and became an avid listener. Lo and behold, men began clamoring for her attention. Later, she was inspired to start a yoga practice and a journal she called, "Cry, Pray, Love."

Fast forward and Genevive is now living with a darling man who reads her poetry and takes her for walks and beautiful trips. While a man's financial situation was never a concern for her, he turned out to be very wealthy. She was drawn to his sense of confidence, and he didn't share his financial status with her, meeting her in the guesthouse attached to his property. It wasn't until he committed to her emotionally that he invited her into his estate home. His life became joy-filled and her life was infused with tenderness. Today she is glowing, and exquisitely and uniquely herself. My prayers are that Elizabeth, like Genevive, will go through the complex and mysterious transition back to herself.

I don't have to wait long to hear good news from David and Elizabeth. One month later, both return with wide smiles.

"We've been working hard, doing our homework, and I think things are better," Elizabeth volunteers. "Man, those hormones are making such a difference. The dead feeling is definitely lifting, and my orgasms are better and stronger. I am using two lozenges of oxytocin rather than one as you prescribed. Is that okay? It really helps."

"Absolutely! There are almost no known side effects to it, except possibly a bit of fatigue if your adrenals are low. Try it when you're going out to an event and notice how much more connected you feel to everyone. It's super safe. How are your other hormones going? Do you still have PMS?"

> *Women's orgasms can take them deeper and deeper into desire, where they literally leave their bodies for hours in one orgasmic wave after the next, each orgasm building more desire, wanting more.*

Elizabeth smiles at David. "My PMS is almost non-existent. I do two clicks of estrogen morning and evening, and I'm using my Kegel machine almost every night. There is definitely a payoff! I think the Dream Cream and the Kegels work great—and oh, my breasts are becoming sensitive. It's almost a problem because they ache a bit."

"Wonderful! I clasp my hands together. "How often are you making love? Do you feel more desire and attraction to David?"

"We are doing great! We're making love twice a week," Elizabeth gleefully responds. "And, yes! I am strangely attracted to his smell and he moves in this sexy way."

"David? Are things okay now?"

"Well," David chuckles, "all this thinking about sex and doing the sexual breath work and yoga practices has unleashed the beast in me, so I could make love with my goddess every day—or even more. This stuff works for men too. I don't feel exactly like I'm twenty, but almost."

"Daviiiiiiid," Elizabeth wails. "I thought we were doing really well."

I reach out and touch her arm. "Now, now, Elizabeth, the tables are easily turned. Once you get super healthy, you will appreciate David being there for you. In fact, women actually have a much larger sensual capacity than men. Do you know that the feminine has an insatiable component to it? Women's orgasms can take them deeper and deeper into desire, to where they literally leave their bodies for hours in one orgasmic wave after the next, each orgasm building more desire, wanting more. It's not like the masculine response, where his desire ceases after an ejaculation."

I think back to my own experience and muse that it is a rare man who knows how to ride these tsunami waves of desire. In fact, men often feel pretty challenged when they experience the insatiable aspects of the feminine. It's not just a woman's sensual side that can be insatiable. Women always seem to want more of everything: more time with their man, more attention, more talk, more intimacy.

"David, can I share a secret with you?" I ask.

"Absolutely! I'm all ears."

I give him my full attention. "Men crave freedom, and because the insatiable feminine needs so much of a man's attention, he often feels controlled by her needs. He then tries to control and contain the feminine aspects of his partner in order to free himself from her control. That is a mistake, however, because the highest freedom for most men is to be taken out of their minds into the passionate, ecstatic realm of Pure Presence and Being. That is authentic freedom."

David nods with understanding.

"That realm is the feminine natural state, and a man's ultimate freedom and regenerative power is found in his union with that feminine shakti energy, ignited by his beloved. It is not going to be a polite, controlled feminine who will take him there. A man kills the golden goose when he tries to control feminine energy, then sadly realizes he has so contained it that his sexual energy is also killed. Uniting with that energy, rather than trying to control it, is ultimately the greatest freedom for a man."

"Oh, my God, I guess that controlling man would be me," David bemoans. "I've been trying to make Elizabeth more reasonable and less emotional as we face problems together. I'm always saying, 'Now, Elizabeth, don't be so emotional; let's be rational.' Or, 'Let's think this through in a calm way.' And then she really isn't uncontrollable like she used to be. But she also isn't as sexy."

> *"Uniting with that energy, rather than trying to control it, is ultimately the greatest freedom for a man."*

He puts his head in his hands. "I killed the golden goose; I have been making her masculine."

"David, dear one, the shakti fire has not gone out in Elizabeth. Look at how sweetly receptive she is to you. She needs your direction when she's this vulnerable and open. Look at her. Take her in and feel the immense love she has for you. The feminine always forgives, and she's already forgiven your lack of understanding. She needs you in order to be her highest unbridled self, just as you need her to become yours." I glance at Elizabeth then back to David. "Besides, it's not just you who did this. Being successful in the masculine workplace will make a woman more masculine. Our entire society tries to control and kill feminine energy; it is threatened by both the regenerative and the destructive nature of it."

As I speak, David and Elizabeth look into each other's eyes and become silently lost in each other. After a few moments, they look back at me with open and receptive gazes. I smile at them. "What you just did, looking into each other's eyes so intently, is a beautiful practice that connects your souls. It's amazing, isn't it?"

"Yes!" they exclaim in unison.

"I suggest you connect like that while talking, eating together, or making love. Simply stop what you are doing and let your eyes make love."

I pause then add, "Elizabeth, I was wondering if David is approaching you in a way that ignites your feminine nature?"

She grimaces. "Well, I have probably shut him down so many times he's probably a bit afraid to approach me as strongly as my feminine nature sometimes desires. I guess I want him to catch me and just take me but …"

"Ahhhh, not to worry. This brings us to David Deida, another tantric master. In one of his classes I took, a man in the audience complained that his woman who didn't respond favorably to his polite and deferential requests to make love. He seemed to be an earnest man but with a compulsive manner about him. After hearing his lengthy complaints spoken, with his longhaired beauty sitting quietly by his side—Deida turned to the audience and asked the women to raise their hands if they would jump into that man's arms if he had approached them in the same manner. Of the hundred women only two responded positively while the others enthusiastically declined the offer. 'Noooo,' 'Ewwww,' 'Icky,' 'Never!'"

Dida responded, "How many of you would like your lover to throw you down and fuck you?" A huge cheer went up from the women, including me.

I lock eyes with David. "What does this mean to you? Do you get this?"

> *"I contend that it is this light ... this divine, loving light that is sensual and extremely alluring."*

A huge smile spreads across his face. "Yeah, I want to do that, but I feel a bit timid because I was getting my balls bitten off for about three years. I'm a respectful guy and I haven't wanted to impose my will on Elizabeth."

I grimace. "I understand. Men have really been messed up, first in the 50s by the silent John Wayne image that shuts them down, then being emasculated in the 60s by the Women's Liberation Movement. Men don't know what to do any more. And poor women! What's a liberated woman, anyway? Is it an exhausted woman trying to do it all: children, a big job, maybe a husband to support, *and* being a sexual diva? Or is it a woman with her body relaxed and flowing, letting light shimmer through her? I contend that it is this light ... this divine, loving light that is sensual and extremely alluring. And it feels really good—wonderful, in fact—to simply be that light."

Elizabeth chimes in. "The young women on my staff have no problem being feminine and using their rather seductive nature to get what they want. I'm learning from them. Women have actually given up a lot of their power by acting like men."

I nod in agreement. "A case in point is my daughter, Beryl, who recently told me about her move from New York back to California. 'Oh, mommy,' she shared with me in front of her boyfriend, John, 'he is magnificent! He figured out the whole trip for us—how to move the cheapest way, where to buy the boxes, and then . . .' she lights up with total joy as she reaches out to caress his face, 'John came over to my apartment and packed everything! He is the most amazing man in the world!'"

Elizabeth giggles a bit and David perks up.

"Well, the liberated woman in me squirmed just the smallest amount, feeling that maybe she wasn't shouldering enough of the work. But the goddess in me smiled in delight. When a woman treats her man like that he responds very favorably, to say the least. A woman might use this form of praise to manipulate her man but at a higher level it cultivates his masculine essence in service to the feminine, resulting in a deeper, more sensual love. In fact, it is appropriate to recognize and adore one's man, both for purely who he is and for the actions he performs for his woman. By this recognition, he becomes more expanded and loving—a true god-man. And what woman doesn't want to make love with this kind of super-confident, expanded, protective, superman?"

I ask Elizabeth if she attended Dawn Cartright's women's immersion last week. She said she didn't have the time, but she and David signed up for Dawn's couples weekend immersion at the Center. Her workshops are fantastic and she will be a great resource for them both. I also give Elizabeth Rori Raye's info: www.havetherelationshipyouwant.com. Her "Love Scripts" and other astute insights on male-female interactions are very helpful.

"So, my lovers," I finish up, "are you doing the yoga practices Mark Whitwell gave you?"

"Yes," they chime together. "And we love them all—the breath work, the yoga, and the time set aside each week for our 'intimate practices.'"

"Good work! Now would you like to try a time-honored shamanic practice? Do you want to try adding a bit of THC from time to time?"

"Marijuana?" David asks inquisitively.

"I don't want to suggest anything distasteful, but THC and other kinds of herbs have been used by Mayan elders and indigenous people in ceremonies throughout human history. It's used as a tool for developing deeper unity and intimacy with life."

Elizabeth shifts in her chair, then crosses her arms over her chest. "I used to smoke in college and I do remember having some life-changing feelings. But with kids in the house we need to set a good example."

"Absolutely. I fully understand your position. As parents we know kids can get into a lot of trouble with drugs, and we have to be mindful about the messages we send. I do believe, however, that when kids see their parents adoring each other it's really good for them. The world would be a different place if the masculine and feminine were not in a constant battle. I've been describing many ways to cultivate this kind of relationship. I'm not suggesting marijuana as a recreational drug. What I am saying is that perhaps it could occasionally be used to help you and David cultivate a deeper ecstatic intimacy."

"Absolutely we want to try it," David interjects. "This is tame. After all we're working in Hollywood where sex is rampant."

"Elizabeth, what about you? Is this against your moral code?"

"My moral code is to be a good mother and a responsible adult." She furrows her brow. "As David said initially, we tried watching soft porn videos and a number of superficial things but nothing worked. We want to stay together and not get divorced like so many of our friends have, which certainly isn't good for the kids." I watch her countenance lighten. "This inward journey you are mentoring us on is working. I'm more loving and patient. Making

> *"People are using all kinds of drugs like Viagra, which can have so many side effects, including heart attacks; whereas marijuana is a natural herb that has been widely studied and used."*

love with David centers me, and I pass that love on to my kids and my co-workers. They see that I'm up to something and have been asking me what's going on. I am not that b-i-t-c-h I used to be so, yes, let's definitely try a bit of herb and see where it takes us."

I offer them both a warm smile. "Marijuana has changed a fair amount since my university days. Pharmacists now tell me it is very specific in terms of its affects. It is legal for medicinal uses like insomnia, migraines, chronic pain, and also for the treatment of sexual dysfunction. Not to imply that there is any dysfunction in either of you (we all chuckle), but that's the medical term for needing sexual improvement. You can get a legal medical marijuana card from a doctor at one of the clinics on Venice Beach, then visit a dispensary and buy a marijuana candy bar, which is better than smoking. Ask the clerk what blend is best for sexual responses, because some of it is specifically made to treat other conditions."

David laughs. "We'll take a walk today and get our cards. I think Elizabeth gets hesitant, which stops her from being more enthusiastic. This is all rather revolutionary of you, Doctor Prudence!"

I glance at both of them. "I think that kind of revolution passed in the sixties, and I don't personally prescribe THC for my patients. I don't want my clinic to come under any scrutiny, but what I'm suggesting is one of marijuana's legitimate medical uses.

WATTIER,
MARIA A

Expires:
5/18/2021

Item barcode number:
35394017276276

Title: Radiant again & forever :
with bioidentical hormones and
other secrets / Prudence Hall, MD
; forewor

Date: Monday, May 10, 2021

People are using all kinds of drugs like Viagra, which can have so many side effects including heart attack, whereas marijuana is a natural herb that has been widely studied and used. Of course not every medicinal treatment is in alignment with individual values, which I'm mentioning because you are exposed to a lot of crazy stuff in Hollywood."

"Hollywood can definitely be a wild place, but what happens in Hollywood stays there," Elizabeth adds with a smile. "Oops, I forgot the paparazzi. We'll see how it works."

I think about how much sexuality and passion are connected to the heart rather than the head. Marijuana can take partners right into their hearts, which is beautiful to experience. It's like entering into a new world for some of my patients, ushering them into deeper intimacy with themselves and their partners. I think about Brian, one of my clients. He told me last week that for him, marriage without great sexual passion just didn't make sense. "If that's the case, why be married at all?" he asked me. I understand all the other reasons to stay together, but a couple that makes love is much more likely to remain united. They shine in a unique, palable way—love made manifesting into the world.

> *"We have to meet each other in order to create the most sexual intimacy."*

I look at David. "Do you know that women need ample time to talk in order to feel intimate? Out of that intimacy arises their sexuality. Men feel intimacy after experiencing sexual passion and actually don't need to talk much. We have to meet each other in the middle to create the deepest sexual intimacy."

"So, it's not just throw her down and be a real man?" David quips.

We all laugh.

"That's a definite! But you also need to give Elizabeth the opportunity to share her heart with you. She also needs you to share verbally with her, telling her you adore her, maintaining eye contact while making love, helping her to go deeper and deeper with you. A wise friend recently told me he always saves 500 words a day to share with his wife, so when he comes home at the end of a day he always sits down with her to really listen and share. He has had a successful, passionate marriage for forty-five years. This seems like a no-brainer, but when men are fatigued they become more silent, and women's brains interpret this as distance and lack of intimacy."

We exchange hugs. Elizabeth and David head out to discuss their diet and then meet Mark Whitwell for a continuation of their yoga.

I don't hear from David and Elizabeth for a number of months, and then receive a sudden email:

Dearest Dr. Prudence,

We are both in the middle of big productions and haven't had the time to come back, but I just spoke with Maryanne, who saw you a few days ago, and I knew I needed to write you.

David and I are madly and passionately in love. There is such freedom in our relationship, where I can tell him anything and he just listens and holds me. He is not trying to control my emotional responses like he used to, and actually encourages me to be exactly as I want to be. And that is driving me wild. I feel so much more alive. Prudence, it happened! The insatiable feminine is back and I am seducing him nonstop. It feels like we are always in the flow of passionate energy and we just want more and more. The kids keep making fun of us and tell us to go to our room, but really, I know they think we are pretty cool.

I wanted you to know how we're doing and also that we are writing a script about our experiences—you are in it! It's a real Hollywood Pink Pill picture and we think it will be snapped up.

I'll come back for my pap and hormone check in March, but didn't want you to feel we fell off the world.

With our love, dear Prudence (Hey, just like the song!)

Elizabeth and David

I sit quietly in my office taking in the letter. They did it! They just grabbed hold of life and did what they needed to do. I feel their happiness, and as I do, my own journey floods back to me. It was a long journey home to my true feminine nature—one that took me years and a divorce after twenty-five years. I laugh to myself—I'm a slow learner compared to my patients!

As I laugh, my heart opens and I suddenly feel the presence of my own beloved man. I am filled with tenderness. He is currently traveling, but I feel no lack. In truth, as I go through my day, I frequently feel I am making love with him no matter where he may be. I have my breath, my mantras and yoga uniting me with my source. I experience no separation between love and me. I am a flower absorbing the rain as it falls. I am in a receptive state, opening into a deeper and deeper quiet.

I love the light of my beloved's mystic eyes meeting mine. His soul's light meets my soul, shining as the heart of divine love the heart of God. I am "that"; he is "that." There is only love and it is everywhere. We are One voice, One breath, One body. One is love. One is peace. One is joy. One is everywhere.

As part of my journey back to myself, I began writing poetry again after many years of silence.

This small poem was written after an intense four-year period of rescuing my heart after my marriage ended. It was a time of developing the vulnerability and courage I needed to love again. Inspired by a volume of 12th century South Indian temple poetry entitled "God On The Hill," each poem poses a question to "God on the hill" while repeating the most important line of the poem.

I Am Dissolving

You have burned the castle gates
and driven the guards from their posts.
Slashing locked doors you search everywhere,
crying my name in the echoing stillness.
Bound and dying, I hear your footsteps fading.
Please don't leave without me.

I am dissolving

Suddenly wood shatters like thunder, and you are here.
Lifting me gently, you weep as you massage my hands,
freeing me with your eyes, your touch; your loving heart.
Everywhere there is light.
Is this your way, God on the hill?

I am dissolving

In your arms, wind stirs the thirsty earth.
Alpine glow splashes a temple with golden hues.
Monsoon rains descend from nowhere and pellet our bodies,
washing away the pain.
As gongs echo in the wild night, we become all things;
the earth, the rain, the night.

I am dissolving

Takeaway:

- Restoring sexual intimacy is a rewarding pursuit for couples who have lost their connection. I have seen relationships flower at every age and every stage of parenting or careers.

- Causes of low sexual functioning arise from all aspects of being human: the physical body, emotional balance and connection to our true spiritual essence.

- Hormones play a large role in our sexual functioning, including restoring a youthful balance of testosterone, adrenal DHEA, estrogen and thyroid.

- Physical muscle tone, correction of vaginal laity, and addressing fatigue are all important factors.

- Physical and emotional practices help restore intimacy.

My prescription for sexual intimacy:

- A daily yoga practice, even for seven or eight minutes a day, grounds the body. I like Mark Whitwell's "I-Promise," which is available as an App.

- Passion for Women: a great herbal supplement to help increase libido

- Kegel exercises, using a Kegel machine or jade balls

- Oxytocin lozenges

- Super Adrenal: 1-2 capsules daily for women; Mega Adrenal: 1 daily for men (Both contain DHEA.)

- The OSHO kundalini meditation (available online)

Chapter 10

The Path of Fulfillment

During my many years of treating patients, I have often seen how living one's true life purpose is a critical factor in creating vibrant, lifelong health and longevity. I was delighted to see research reviewed in *The Atlantic* addressing exactly this aspect of health. Researchers found that people living their true life purpose live longer and more vibrant lives. They also suffer from fewer strokes and heart attacks, less diabetes, metastatic cancer, neurodegenerative diseases and viral sickness.

> *It is not your chronological age that matters; it is your biological age, and that number is directly connected to your cellular health, but also your emotions, thoughts and connection to your soul's journey.*

The fact is, only one-third of baby boomers or generation X-ers love their work while the other two-thirds are "not engaged" or are downright unhappy with their jobs. My clients confide that with forty or fifty years of life still left, the activities they once loved are no longer available or no longer interest them. Their children are grown; careers have reached their pinnacle; and relationships are less rewarding. I have often seen how the second half of life can be a downward slippery slope of loss: lost dreams, lost love, and lost health. Because so many of my clients suffer this way, I am interested in helping them address "what's next" in life as a valid medical concern.

If this feeling of loss is happening to you, it means you are ready to shed old values and habitual patterns that no longer serve you. It's time to go into the realm of your imagination to create a new life. This needs to be done throughout various stages in life in order to maintain the vital, youthful enthusiasm that connects us to living fully. It's not your chronological age that matters; it is your biological age, and that number is connected directly to your cellular health, your emotions, thoughts, and your soul's journey.

After resourcing, guiding, and mentoring clients for years on what this process entails, I realized it truly does take a community to support and cheer one another on. Out of this need, I created a program called The Path of Fulfillment. This is the mission of the program:

The Path of Fulfillment is The Hall Center's ongoing series of lectures, workshops and individual sessions dedicated to helping you identify and live your life's true purpose. It guides you in developing fulfilling meditative and spiritual practices for lifelong vibrant health and emotional joy, and helps navigate life's challenging transitions in your relationships, careers, and health.

In this chapter we will follow my patient Emily as she searches for and finds her life's purpose. I will also share some of the struggles and insights I encountered on my path as a doctor, and the stories of two of my dearest friends, Karina Stewart and Doron Libshtein. It is my hope that as you follow our struggles and successes, your inner path and purpose will become more clear, helping you manifest your highest, most fulfilling life and vibrant health.

Emily arrives for her six-month appointment and seems unhappy. "Prudence, I don't know what's happening to me. I feel so tired and I don't wake up with enthusiasm any more. God, I might be a bit depressed but there is absolutely no reason for this. I guess I don't feel the highlight of my life should be having lunch with my friends—it feels too shallow. In fact, I don't seem to like my friends that much anymore. Something is lacking. I just don't know what I'm supposed to be doing with my life."

I ask her a few questions and she replies, "My marriage is fine. Peter is great, but he's really getting concerned about me. No problem with the kids—they are super-good but don't need me much. Adam is in college and Jenn is seventeen. She's become my teacher in many ways—it's so bizarre. You got me through my awful menopause and now I feel great physically. But this feels like I'm in another kind of crisis. I just can't put my finger on it. Should I go on antidepressants?"

I carefully look at her hormone levels. I have been balancing her menopausal hormones for almost seven years, and they are all at excellent levels, even her adrenals. Low adrenals can cause a woman to feel like life is passing her by, as can perimenopause or menopause. Low thyroid conditions can too. But none of these apply to Emily.

"Emily my dear, you are fifty-five, and this angst does not appear to be a case of physical imbalance. The parasites you had are gone and your digestive tract is restored. The small amounts of mercury and lead you had have been removed. I know your diet is super and you have never had a problem sleeping. So my answer is no, you should definitely not go on an antidepressant.

"I frequently see this kind of unhappiness when my patients are at a midlife point. For many women it is actually part of their menopausal transition. Women in menopause can feel so tired and sick that they operate only in survival mode. When they get their energy back many feel their lives no longer have much meaning. They ask, 'Is this all there is?' Perhaps this is happening to you, Emily? Do you need to redefine yourself a bit?"

Emily bursts into tears. "Prudence, that's all I think about. What used to interest me in my thirties and forties doesn't interest me now, and I don't have any idea what to do. I keep going over and over in my mind what I should do next. I just don't know, and I am becoming more and more unhappy, feeling I am not where I need to be. Something is missing. I feel I'm meant to do something creative, or somehow help the world, but . . ." She wipes her nose with Kleenex and looks at me with forlorn eyes. "I don't seem to be able to figure it out. I feel lost."

> *To know yourself is not an easy thing, and sometimes crossing off a not-that list will take you to the truth of what really is.*

"Emily, I am so sorry. 'Lost' sounds scary but I have another way of looking at it. Rather than lost, is it possible you are on a journey where the destination hasn't yet been revealed? Perhaps everything you've done up until now has prepared you for a new chapter in your life, but you just haven't discovered it yet."

She sniffs and lets out a deep breath. "I guess I know myself better now than I ever have, but what keeps coming up is all the things I *don't* like and *don't* want to do, not what I could be doing. It feels very negative."

"To know yourself is not an easy thing, and sometimes crossing off a 'not-that' list will take you to the truth of what really is. But it can also create negativity. Coming from a place of gratitude is actually a better way of approaching this dilemma."

"Oh, Prudence, I have become so negative, and I really have so much to be grateful for!"

"Okay, let's go over what comes to mind in terms of what you can be thankful for."

Emily sucks air into her lungs and spills out quick responses. "I am grateful for my health and how quickly you helped me with my horrible menopause. I am so grateful for my husband, whom I really love, and my kids who are healthy and smart. I am grateful for my neighbor who is a mentor to me. I am grateful for my vacations and for my friends at work. But I'm so tired of what I am doing. Oops, I'm getting negative again. I guess I could go wider and say I am grateful we're not at war like so much of the world. I feel safe. I can wear what I want and don't have to cover up like some cultural customs require. I am not enslaved like so many women are. Really, I am grateful for so many things like having a home, food, a car, beautiful weather in Los Angeles ..." A slight smile appears on her lips and she looks at me with hope.

I touch her hand. "See how being grateful changes the energy around us? Everything is a reflection of what is happening inside us. We change our reality by changing our thoughts, emotions, and past conditioning. We are actually changing our very DNA when we change how we operate. Does this make sense?"

Emily ponders my words for a few moments. "Yes, I do need to take responsibility for my life. I slip into feeling like a victim so easily. I took the Landmark Worldwide when I was thirty, and one thing I promised myself was that I wouldn't be a victim in my life. My upbringing with my alcoholic dad makes it easy to do that."

"Landmark Worldwide is a wonderful program, isn't it? It's a perfect place to start in terms of being creators of our lives. I took a number of their classes years ago, which helped me identify and eliminate some of my limiting beliefs. I totally agree that when we take full responsibility for ourselves, it becomes a new way of operating."

Emily nods. "It was important for me to take that class, but I seem to have forgotten. I don't know what to do."

"That's why I started The Path of Fulfillment at the Center. Do you know about it?"

"No, but it sounds like I need to." She nods vigorously. "What is it?"

"It consists of the workshops and individual sessions we offer at the Center. Health includes not just the physical body but also our emotions, thoughts, and our connection to our soul's purpose. The Path of Fulfillment program helps each of us live our most expanded, conscious, and fulfilling life. I'm surprised you haven't come to any of our events."

"I always get your emails, and the people you bring in seem so interesting. I guess I wasn't aware what it was really about. I should have been going."

Many of my clients echo Emily's words and I offer her a warm smile. "Things happen when the timing is right. Besides, we offer workshops all the time. I created the program because I have been on my own path for many years and I know how important it has been for me to have mentors. I want to assist people who, like you and me, are looking for fulfillment and purpose in life. It's part of True Health."

As thoughts of my own journey flash through my mind, I hear Emily saying, "God, Prudence, just the idea of being on a path is a new concept. I mean, I have viewed my life as a series of accomplishments that haven't led me anywhere. Do you really think there's a unique path each of us follow?"

"I can absolutely and resoundingly say yes, there is a path. It begins with who you are and what you love—your talents and strengths. Like the story of blind men describing an elephant by the parts they touch, each Path of Fulfillment teacher offers a different way to come back to yourself. Want to give it a try?"

"I have the need and the time. *I am ready!*" she blurts out.

"Excellent. Whenever I hear the words 'I'm ready' in the context of beginning an epic journey, I always recall the poet David

Whyte. Have you heard his poem about the salmon being ready to go on its journey back to the sea?"

"I don't know who David is, but I'd like to hear his poem."

"Good. I'll download his 'Song for the Salmon' poem for you before you leave. It's the perfect poem to have as you start your journey home to yourself. David's poetry has inspired me over the years and I often listen to his tapes on long drives. If you like the salmon poem, you'll love his CD collection, 'Clear Mind, Wild Heart.'"

I glance up at the clock and realize I have spent almost forty minutes with Emily and am getting behind with my other patients. "I'll connect you to a few of our teachers so you can see who resonates with you. And I'll see you at some of our workshops—I attend whenever I can."

I hug Emily and walk her to the door. She looks at me with hope and new resolve.

I next see Emily two months later at Jeffrey Van Dyk's workshop and greet her warmly.

"Prudence, I told you I was starting my journey! In fact, I am well into it. I've been working with Jeffrey every month. Did he tell you?"

I smile because Emily's name has come up several times. "I know a bit, but not everything—just that he is mentoring you and you are buzzing into action."

"Well, my life is much sweeter—like that young salmon David wrote about."

I throw back my head and laugh. "We are that salmon indeed, Emily, being called on an epic journey back to the wild sea."

"Jeffrey and I started with exploring who I am. That took quite a while, because I have had a lot of emotional trauma stopping me from connecting to myself. He helped me see how the trauma was actually my PhD for the next phase of life. I wasn't aware that I'm an artist at heart. I'm moved by beauty and love beautiful creations, which is why I loved David's poem."

"That is wonderful, Emily. I didn't know that about you."

"Well, I had forgotten about the creative me … and Prudence, next we did a meditation about the life I see myself living. He helped me become more emotional about that vision, and now those emotions are driving me forward. I'm trying to act like I'm already living the life I dreamed of having. Focus and passion are how I'm catching what I need to do to get there. It can feel bizarre and at times like I am Alice in Wonderland, but I'm doing it."

"Wow, Emily, you have certainly been a good student!"

"Yes I am!" she says and laughs. "And I took Doron Libshtein's 'Walk Your Path' class and created my 'Ideal Calendar.' I'm putting some of the things I love back into my life. It's super easy and inspiring."

"Cool, Emily. I'm working on my calendar too. Doron is a wonderful mentor, isn't he?"

It is amazing to see how much life beams from her eyes.

"Yes he is! And Jeffrey tells me I need to surround myself with people who meet me at a higher vibration while detaching myself from those who don't. That's why I also work with Doron and why I'm here today. I realized a lot of my old friends weren't on the same path I'm on. It was great while we were raising our kids, but now we don't have much in common. The thing is, I didn't know I was on a path, so I felt confused. That got cleared up almost immediately, because focusing is sharp and exacting. I'm also in Jeffrey's 'genius' group once a month and we support one another, which is why we're all here tonight." She laughs and I feel a deep connection with her.

A tall man comes over and hugs Emily. He has an enchanting accent and it turns out he's in her group. I greet Miguel and leave them to their excited talk. I'm so happy Emily is on her path with such excellent guidance. Without a supportive community it can feel pretty dark at times.

Eight months later I look at my schedule and see Emily's name. At her appointed time, she marches into my office and plops down on my couch, looking amazingly fit. She has a beautiful light about her.

I greet her warmly. "How are you, you wonder woman?"

She tells me she has come in to make sure her hormones are all balanced, which she is quite sure they are. She's right—almost everything is perfect.

"How've you been?"

She smiles mischievously. "Didn't you wonder if I was okay?"

I laugh. "I knew you were great! I felt it and knew it, but catch me up."

"I have crossed many seas and had so many adventures you can't imagine. I have learned who I am, and I'm in love—madly!" She laughs. "I'm in love with myself, and I found I have a writer in me. I've written a book about my journey, and I feel this is only my first step because I know there are more parts to the puzzle."

"Really? Amazing! I am so happy for you and I can't wait to read it." I pause and look at her. "I bet it will help others with their own path."

"Exactly. It's a little like *Eat, Pray, Love*. Bless Julia Roberts for playing that part, which helped me define myself and my path.

"You know Jeffrey. As he mentored me, I saw what I needed and who my tribe is. I have wonderful friends and I'm doing things I never would have imagined possible. I have actually become an avid mountaineer and I'm hiking with my tribe through the most beautiful countries in the world. I started with a hike around Mont Blanc, and have been to three other countries since then. My kids love my trips and have come on a few of them when they aren't in school."

"This is so beautiful, Emily. I am happy for you! I love to hike too and maybe will be able to join you one day. I'd love to hike in the Himalayas."

Emily searches my face. "I would go back there. It's a beautiful part of the world. And I would love you to write a few lines for the book cover. Could you possibly . . ."

"With pleasure! I will read it and already know I'll be inspired."

"Truly thank you, Prudence. I am so happy to have your endorsement and will email you the script—and I do feel the Himalayas are the ultimate inspiration. Hiking amongst those towering mountains was the best!"

After making a few adjustments in her health routine, we hug warmly then walk to the door where Wendy is waiting to refill Emily's hormones. I marvel at the change in Emily. No depression, irritability or fatigue. She is radiant and full of life.

In sharing with you how Emily broke through into greater self-understanding and life purpose, I am cast into some of the defining moments of my own life path. How did I decide that becoming a doctor was the right choice? How did I stay on track with my dreams and not let them slip away? Throughout my life I was always called a "tender heart," because I never killed ants or other insects. I would rush to save them, fight with the person who was trying to kill them, and gently take them outside. I tended injured animals and also had a kind of sixth sense about what people needed, along with a desire to help them. I knew I had a scientific mind as well as a tender heart, because I loved learning about nature, astronomy and geology.

One day, however, I encountered a harsh and nasty side of science. A baby bird had fallen out of its nest and I rushed it to my favorite science teacher to help me save it. I was in eighth grade and loved this teacher. Under his tutelage I was becoming a young scientist and the best student in the class. When he saw the bird, he agreed to help save it and rushed with it to the back room. Then he returned without it. I was puzzled and asked him what the bird needed. He told me he had immediately killed it because there was no way it could survive, that he was doing the bird a favor. I was heartbroken, furious and *knew* beyond any doubt that we could have saved it. In my outrage I swore I would never again involve myself with heartless science. And I didn't for many years.

When I was in high school, I lived in Spain and later in France. I had a strong desire to help humanity but wasn't sure what field or how to proceed. I eventually enrolled at the University of Toulouse, where I studied International Relations. As I studied the plight of poor women in developing nations, I knew I wanted to help all women in some meaningful way. Even though I was disillusioned with science, some of my French friends were medical students. I caught myself fantasizing, *If only I were a doctor. I would work in developing countries to help poor women.* This desire grew within me until I finally gave in and decided to give science another try. After all, I needed it to become a doctor.

When I shared this dream with my father, a founding Provost at the University of California Santa Cruz, he scoffed. "No way you'd ever get into medical school. I counsel those premed kids all the time and they are super smart. Besides, you haven't taken any science classes. Prudy, (only my father got to call me that) you're a renaissance person; med school won't work for you."

Doubt seized me. Maybe he was right. He knew everything about university acceptance criteria, and he certainly knew me. And yes, students were always saying how impossible it was to get into medical school. Yet it was impossible to forget what I now knew: I knew that being a doctor was right for me, and I knew it deep within me. I considered that my father might not be speaking about me, but instead about his own life. Or perhaps he was trying to save me from the bitterness of not achieving my dreams. Regardless of his motivations, I knew I needed to rely on myself and figure this all out.

With dreams of medical school in my heart, I left France to attend the University of California Santa Cruz. I married my French-Spaniard aristocratic boyfriend and took my first biology class in six years. I told myself that if I did poorly I would give up my dream of being a doctor. In that first premed class, I was overwhelmed by the competitiveness of the students and how hard they studied. Maybe my father was right, maybe I couldn't do it. Maybe I didn't have it in me. But when I received my first biology grade, I was stunned when I realized I was the top student in the class. I was relieved, breathless, and filled with new resolve. If I could succeed in one class, I could do so in all of them. I started "seeing" myself as a doctor. I envisioned myself succeeding, graduating, and helping thousands of women. I reached deep inside and became the most stubborn,

> *I started "seeing" myself as a doctor. I envisioned myself succeeding and graduating and helping thousands of women.*

willful person who had ever lived. Nothing or no one could stop my dream from coming true. I didn't hang around people who would say that medical school was too hard to get into, or that only smart people got in. I may not be the smartest, but I also knew I'd be a fantastic doctor.

My fellow students didn't share this attitude. They complained about the classes, the difficulty of getting into medical school, and talked incessantly about the people who had failed. Maybe it was true for others, but it wasn't true in my case. For me, not only did I *know* I'd get into medical school, I knew I would do so *immediately*.

After one year of science classes, with still another year of premed left, I decided to apply to a single medical school as a way of testing the application process. I chose UC Berkeley, because they had an innovative medical school with a big mission about being of service. By this time my father was impressed with my successes in premed classes and felt I had a fighting chance of getting into medical school. I went to him and said, "Daddy, I'm putting in my first application and need just the right quote to open my essay with—a quote that encapsulates who I am and why I would make a good doctor. I know you'll have the perfect one." He thought for no more than ten seconds and spontaneously quoted Bertrand Russell:

"Three passions, simple but overwhelmingly strong have governed my life: the longing for love, the search for knowledge, and unbearable pity for the suffering of mankind."

"This is you, Prudy," he said. "This is exactly who you are. This will do the trick."

I carefully filled out the application, putting all my hopes and dreams into the essay, as well as the Bertrand Russell quote. I was astonished when UC Berkeley called me for an interview. They asked if I wanted six individual interviews or to meet all six interviewers at once. A voice that sounded much like mine said, "Six all at once would be great." *Was that really me?* I was close to being terrified!

On the appointed day, I intuitively grabbed a bunch of treats and threw them in a basket. I jumped in the car and drove from Santa Cruz to UC Berkeley. I still remember the blue dress I wore that matched the pristine blue sky. It was one of the dresses I used to wear in France and I felt a subtle transformation from the casual Santa Cruz student I had become back to the sophisticated European woman I used to be. I also felt a little like Dorothy on her way to meet the Wizard of Oz. I was introduced to six professors, all men, and all looking rather serious. We decided to sit outside on the lawn because it was a glorious day.

Our formal "scary" interview rapidly became an exciting, animated dialogue and feast. I overflowed with questions and ideas, asking for their input on how I should best proceed with

> *My heart broke into deep sobs of gratitude. My life's purpose was being granted to me.*

my plan to become a gynecologist so that I could help women worldwide. We talked about the highlights and disappointments of their own lives, and how I should approach my career. We munched sandwiches, drank lemonade and devoured all the brownies I had bought—all in a never ceasing dialogue of wonder. It was such a joy to be out of the classroom and talking with people who had already done what I was going to do! Up to this point, I hadn't had any contact with real doctors.

The admissions director came out several times to tell us the interview was over, but we just couldn't stop sharing. Finally, after two hours, we acquiesced and went inside. A kind of enchantment lifted as we saw the anxious faces of the other waiting students. I slowly drove home, lost in the moments we had shared and the excitement of my future life. I was touched by the commitment of each doctor and how each one had used their degree in a different way. I also had a better understanding of what it would take to embark on the difficult and intensive path of becoming a doctor. They told me about the enormous number of hours and long years of grueling work they had endured. I knew I could do it as well, and knew with certainty that all I needed was for the red flag to drop.

I heard nothing from UC Berkeley after the interview and was soon immersed in the next semester with mind-numbing hours of work. I assumed I was not accepted. How could I with so many classes left to take? Several months later I was surprised to receive a thin envelope from UC Berkeley. It was way too thin to be an acceptance letter, but as I held it, I remembered our time on the lawn together and felt a brief flicker of hope that maybe, just maybe . . .

It was a spring day with the sky exploding in violet-blue and the campus hills alive with vibrant smells of dry grass and redwood trees. I carefully opened the one page letter and, as I did, I saw the small words that changed my life forever: "Congratulations, you have been accepted to UC Berkley."

My heart broke into deep sobs of gratitude. My life's purpose was being granted to me. I had not been wrong in this deep knowing and inner recognition of who I was. I would be a doctor! I would be a doctor, the ultimate privilege. My heart flew open, filling with profound joy. I thanked the professors who had supported me and celebrated with my family. I signed up to take the remaining core classes in summer school and prepared for my new life in Berkeley with my French husband.

Over the next eight years, I trained first at UC Berkeley and then at USC, caring for the sickest and poorest members of our society. Exhausted, frequently wearing bloodstained surgical scrubs, I worked day and night providing urgent and emergency care. I kept reminding myself that 80 percent of success comes from simply showing up, so I steadfastly showed up for each patient. I suffered greatly with the pain of my patients and with all the misery and poverty I saw. In the darkened hospital halls at night, when I found a few minutes of solitude, I knew that only grace allowed me to be the doctor rather than the patient. My work with my sick and dying patients became a kind of non-ending meditation and initiation into the depths of human pain.

> *Suffering is not the way. Love is the way.*

One night in the stillness of the darkened hospital, crushed by fatigue, I felt overwhelming despair and sadness. Who had I become? Crying for my patients and despairing for humanity I was exhausted beyond physical endurance. In a true dark night of the soul, I reviewed the decisions that had brought me to this place of desolation. I saw how, in my longing to be an excellent doctor, I had forgotten the tenderhearted healer who saved animals. I saw that by embracing Western medicine I had dismissed the mystical parts of humanity I had always known. I saw how quickly I slipped into suffering and how unhappy and alone I felt. "Please help me," I murmured.

Suddenly, I felt my suffering lift a little. I felt less tired as I remembered the dream I had worked so hard to achieve. I saw with clarity that the dream I had yearned for was the dream I was actually living. This was what my living my dream looked like and really, it wasn't so bad. It was actually fascinating to be learning so much. My heart filled with respect and appreciation for the mission I had chosen. Tears of love replaced my tears of pain. I suddenly felt love for all humanity.

In that moment I knew one of the important truths of my life: *suffering is not the way.* No matter how much compassion or understanding suffering might create, it is not nearly as transformative or powerful as love. *Love is the way.* Love is all there is. I no longer needed to suffer. My suffering was not good for my patients and it wasn't good for me. All I had to do was love. And with this realization, I identified my true life's purpose. My purpose was to be Pure Love, bringing more and more Light and Love into the world. Medicine was simply a tool for doing so.

Two of my dearest friends, Karina Stewart and Doron Libshtein, have also been on powerful paths to living their unique life purposes. How did they identify what they felt most passionate about, and how did they then create a lifelong mission from it? I feel their stories are important to share, because both are intimately involved in the life purpose they created for themselves. Their purposes are bigger than life, and certainly bigger than each of them is. I want you to take all three of our stories and let them help you see your own path and purpose more clearly. I want you to dream big, and like Karina and Doron who never gave up, I don't want you to give up on your dreams either.

Karina Stewart has passed through both hard and miraculous times on her magnificent life path. She told me this story about creating Kamalaya with her husband John Stewart. Kamalaya is the premier wellness resort in the world—not only for detox/cleanses, but for stress relief, natural healing, and personal transformation.

Karina Stewart's Path

Prudence: Was there any juncture in your life where you could have played small, rather than continue on your own path?

Karina: Yes, the one that comes to my mind very strongly is when I was living in Seattle after I had graduated from Princeton. I earned a BA in cultural anthropology, which is not the most practical degree, and I was taking a break because I didn't want to enroll in graduate school until I was absolutely clear about what I wanted to do. The expectation was to just keep going and get another degree, but I didn't exactly know what direction was right. I had sent my GRE's off to random universities, and Stanford was trying to recruit me for their MBA program; but that was not where my interests lay. It made sense: a BA from Princeton and an MBA from Stanford, and blah, blah, blah. I could feel the part of me that wanted to fulfill society's expectation, and in some very unconscious ways also fulfill my mother's thwarted, truncated love of learning. I could feel that pull.

Well, right at that decision-making time, I was exposed to Taoism. I met a Taoist teacher, Master Dao Shun Ni, and I invited him to give a little talk. I thought maybe 30-40 people would show up but more than 250 people signed up and we had to move to a big auditorium. During that evening it felt like he was speaking directly to me—like there was no one else in the room.

"Some people go through life," he said, "fulfilling the expectations of others—of their families, of society—obtaining all the right degrees and certificates and awards to hang on the wall. Other people decide to follow their"—he didn't say 'passion,' he said 'their calling'—and take the path less traveled." I couldn't believe he was inside my head, talking specifically to me.

At that point I had an ah-ha moment and in that exact instant turned away from the expectations and seals of approval from my family and society. I decided not to go to Stanford, and instead to enroll in Chinese medical school. It was a fulfillment of my passion and what I had actually longed to do, but had suppressed. I moved from Seattle to Santa Monica and attended Dr. Ni's acupuncture school. Acupuncture was not well known in the US at that time, and all my Princeton friends were shocked saying things like, "What? Chinese medicine? Are you kidding? If you're interested in medicine, why not do the real thing and go to medical school?"

Even my close friends gave me flak and incredibly, even the Western medical doctors at the Chinese school also questioned

> *The end result is to inspire, educate and guide people to go further into their own journey of transformation.*

why I didn't go to a "regular" medical school. Everyone thought I did it because I couldn't do the real thing. What they didn't understand was my true motivation. My life had changed in ways I would never, ever exchange.

Prudence: Where did this choice take you?

Karina: To Kamalaya! I never could have envisioned or started Kamalaya without this training. Everything I learned in Chinese medical school eventually led me to create Kamalaya with my husband, John.

Prudence: Did your Taoist path take you first to India, and then Nepal?

Karina: Yes, it did, and of course I had my Indian teacher while I was still at Princeton and spent as much time as I could with him in India over a number of years. So I had regularly travelled to India. It was actually my husband John who took me to Nepal. When he asked me if I'd be willing to live in Nepal, I was already very interested in continuing my studies in China, so I was open to his suggestion. I said, "Absolutely."

In Nepal, I had a friend who studied Chi Gong, one who did Ayurveda massage, one who did Ayurveda cuisine, and another who was a yoga master. So I had already started pulling together a network and could envision how we could work together. I started looking for a building in Nepal where I could bring this whole concept together, including a café and everything. And then we found land outside of Katmandu with partners. But my husband, who traveled extensively as an Asian Art antiquities collector, stumbled on land in Thailand, which he fell in love with. That is where we ultimately built Kamalaya.

Prudence: Tell us what Kamalaya is and what it stands for.

Karina: Kamalaya is a retreat center for transformation of the body, mind, spirit, and emotions—the whole package. We create an environment for people to awaken and deepen while on their soul-path, whether they are beginners or have been on their path for a long time. The entry point can be their body, emotions, or the energetic realm through meditation. It doesn't matter which portal because the end result is to inspire, educate, and guide people to go further into their own journey of transformation.

Prudence: And it is an award-winning, world-class . . .

Karina: Yes, it's a multi award-winning resort that has received wide recognition in the industry for having set a new benchmark for what is possible.

Prudence: And you are the spokesperson and cofounder . . .

Karina: My husband and I are the founders, and I work very closely with the wellness director, the chef, and the marketing team. I am considered the face of Kamalaya, the spokesperson, the worldwide educator. I am delighted that John is now taking on that role as well.

Prudence: And this came out of your choice to follow your unique path?

Karina: Absolutely! It was the critical turning point I described. I would have created something else but not the unique emanation of my heart that is Kamalaya. I say unique because I had the courage to take the path less traveled—the path of my heart. And the amazing thing is that everything I have learned from Kamalaya feels like it is beginning to take me on another creative journey. I am ready and waiting for my next step to unfold.

Prudence: Thank you, dear Karina! I know the courage it took to create Kamalaya with John, and I can't wait to see what comes next as you follow the path of your loving heart.

I take Karina to the airport after our discussion, remembering how we met in Bali those many years ago, and have been treasured friends for all these years. We have referred patients back and forth, been on retreats together and are inspired by who the other is being and continually becoming.

Doron Libshtein is another courageous and inspiring creator of his life and journey. My relationship with Doron begin with him becoming my mentor. It soon developed into a precious friendship and Doron taking on the position as the Center's chairman. A world leader in self-development, Doron is a mentor to the world's top mentors, an author, and strategic entrepreneur in the area of personal growth.

In his lectures, Doron frequently tells the story of how his life transformation has taken him to a very different place than he ever would have imagined—a mission of connecting world leaders for global transformation.

Doron Libshtein's Path

Prudence: Welcome Doron. I am so pleased you agreed to speak to us about how you discovered your life's purpose. Could you start by describing your early life?

> *When I was instructed to write out my life vision, the words spontaneously and instantaneously came to me: "Bring coaching to the masses."*

Doron: Well, I was raised in Israel, the oldest of five children. We remain a close and supportive family. After secondary school I joined the army for four years. When I finished at age twenty-two, I started my career at Microsoft in a junior position. While there, I received my university degree and MBA, which helped me rapidly progress. When I left Microsoft after fourteen years, I was a senior director in Europe, responsible for 4,000 employees, four billion dollars, and four teams in different countries. During my career at Microsoft, I was also VP of Marketing in Israel, and the founder and CEO of MSN, the Microsoft network in Israel. So I had a full career at Microsoft.

Prudence: Were you satisfied and happy with what you were doing at Microsoft?

Doron: I absolutely loved what I did. I was very involved on every level and felt I was doing what I was meant to do. It was a highly responsible job and, as seen by society, the pinnacle of success. From the moment I became a manager in 1996, I was mentored for the next eleven years by Microsoft executives. Because this was so beneficial to my own growth, it became the way I also managed my own teams. In my role at Microsoft Euro, I traveled between countries supporting my top managers. I was their mentor, their coach, and I loved it.

Prudence: Was mentoring a successful strategy with your employees?

Doron: Yes. The first year in Microsoft Euro, 2003, we won the Best Team Award. I credit this to the fact that the first thing I did when I arrived in London was to hire a company called "Culture Shock" to coach my British team to work effectively with other cultures. You couldn't imagine for example, how differently the Dutch and Brits approach the same problem, so I taught my team and myself to be very effective across many cultures.

A year later, I decided to take coaching classes to expand my skills. When I signed up I received passes to see Tony Robbins speak. He was amazing—speaking to 15,000 people and at the same time directly to me. When I was instructed to write out my life vision, the words spontaneously and instantaneously came to me: "Bring coaching to the masses."

Prudence: Was this a turning point in your career?

Doron: It was a turning point in my life, but I didn't know it yet. I was in the middle of my career at Microsoft and certainly not thinking of leaving. I interpreted the life vision message as meaning to bring coaching to all 4,000 of my employees and Microsoft clients, not just my top managers. In other words I thought this was the fulfillment of the Microsoft vision, which was to enable people and businesses to realize their full potential.

I presented several proposals to top U.S. Microsoft management, including an online less costly version, but my proposal was turned down. However, I was so inspired by the vision itself that I couldn't give it up—it was burning within me. I just had to do it! I was sorry not to fulfill it with Microsoft, but now I had the opportunity to do it for myself. So I asked my brother to start a business, which we later named Mentors Channel. I made plans to leave Microsoft within a year so I could join the company and bring mentoring to all people, uniting the spiritual with the physical to help shift the collective global consciousness.

Prudence: What did people say about you leaving Microsoft?

Doron: They were in complete shock and thought I was insane! I was at the top of my career—the youngest Israeli to be in such a powerful position. No one believed I was going to do this. They felt that Microsoft and I were "one," so everyone tried to convince me to stay. It wasn't easy. I knew, however, that if I didn't implement this vision, my life would not be fulfilled. In fact, I felt that everything I had learned up to this point had prepared me to be successful in this expansive vision.

Prudence: Looking back, how did your vision untold?

Doron: This is where I surprised myself. I thought that just like most other aspect of my life it would go smoothly—that with a high consciousness and purposeful company everything I envisioned would easily manifest. However, the first six years were very, very tough years—years where I spent all of my savings on this visionary business, and then needed to sell my house to continue funding our operations. There were times when I questioned everything about what we were doing.

Even though I brought in top mentors of the world to partner with me, I just couldn't find the formulas to fulfill my vision. I spent almost six years and three phases where I changed many aspects of the business. Still I never deviated from the vision of contributing to the shift in global consciousness through mentoring.

Prudence: Did you ever consider dropping the company to do something else?

Doron: No! I never considered that even when I sold assets and use my retirement savings to keep it going; even when I needed to take on other opportunities as chairman of other companies to keep afloat. Many of my friends would say, "Listen, Doron, you've hit the wall so many times that you'd better give up. Admit that you belong to the big companies, and go back to them. Make a fortune, enjoy life, and put this drama aside."

Prudence: So why didn't you do that? What stopped you from doing what most people would consider a wise thing to do?

Doron: It was a deep knowing within me that, no matter what other people said, this was my true purpose in life. This is what I would bring to the world and would be the fulfillment of my life path. I *knew* it would be successful. I saw that each time I overcame an obstacle, the company reached a higher frequency, going from thousands, to tens of thousands, and eventually to millions of people.

Prudence: Now that you have millions of people and very successful programs, how do you feel about it?

Doron: Yes, we reach hundreds of millions of people through our Facebook community, and millions with our programs, and I feel it is only the beginning. I see our company touching 500 million people, uniting with other companies in this industry to work together to bring a higher consciousness to the world. I am partnering with The Hall Center, I Amplify, Wild Divine and other organizations around the world. As well, I want our WellBE wearable stress bracelet to help reduce stress worldwide, and our Israeli-Arab team to help promote global peace.

Prudence: That is truly inspiring.

Doron: I feel inspired too, and this state of knowing keeps me walking my own path. That's why I created my newest program, "Walk Your Path." It is not really about the goals or about the wins. Those are the gifts that you collect by being on your authentic path. It is all about staying on your path, knowing "this is what I must do," and then doing it.

Prudence: Mentors Channel has been one of your biggest teachers, hasn't it?

> *The first thing I'd say is dream, dream, dream!*

Doron: Absolutely. Because of Mentors Channel I have been fortunate to work with the top mentors in the world and directly experience them through their courses, books, and having quality time with them. I've spent many, many days with my mentors through which I've built the capacity within me to take this work of consciousness to countless people.

Prudence: What's the next step?

Doron: I'm glad to say that I'm starting to become a teacher myself after mentoring for the last twenty-five years. A mentor guides others through their own life experiences. Whereas a teacher offers universal wisdom and knowledge to his students.

Prudence: Those who know you recognize you as an inspirational teacher and leader. I understand you are forming a worldwide alliance to accelerate the evolution of global consciousness.

Doron: Yes, and the message I'm getting from my alliances is that we share a similar mission and vision. So we are reconnecting and fulfilling our shared mission to transform the world in all areas. We do it in the health industry,

> *When you have a big dream, never give up.*

in the consciousness raising industry and any other area—there is so much to do. And this is what you do in your industry too,

Prudence. You are a leader in your industry, and this is what we do together. We help transform the world to a healthier, balanced, "natural" state.

Prudence: Yes, this is what we are blessed and privileged to do. In closing, do you have any advice for anyone starting out on their own path?

Doron: Of course, of course! The first thing I'd say is dream, dream, dream! It is so important to dream. Most of us live small, and we deserve to live big lives. So being on the Path of Fulfillment starts with big dreams. I suggest spending time just imagining what you *want* to do. Really invest time in exploring this. Ask yourself, "Who am I? What gifts do I bring to the world? What is my mission?" With that beginning, each individual can move on to the fulfillment of their vision. In business, what we call "planning" is an important next step. Planning is the combination of dreaming and imagining, which births an inspired plan of action.

The next thing I would love to share is that when you have a big dream, *never* give up. You never know if you are only thirty centimeters from your goal. If you are facing some difficulties or experiencing challenges, this means there's a reason why you need extra time. Stick with what you inwardly know until it becomes your reality. Have a big dream, focus your thoughts on that dream; plan wisely and imagine you are already living that dream.

> *Success is staying authentically on our path, knowing that whatever will come is there for a reason.*

My third message is this: Success is staying on our authentic path. By staying on our path, we experience life in its fullness. The challenges and great achievements are both equally part of the process. So with that, I seek to inspire entrepreneurs and seekers to continue on their journey, bringing innovation and new light to the world, and bringing a collective consciousness for global transformation. This is the journey: from Me, to We, to One.

Prudence: Thank you, Doron, for inspiring and sharing with us the ways in which you have followed your heart's knowing.

I have loved writing this chapter! I loved it because, unlike the previous chapters, it addresses the aspect of health that inspires me the most. Vital health means being strong and free of diseases and contributes to living a long life. No one wants to have long, miserable years of living. It is about having vital health and being enthusiastic and joyful in our lives.

Interestingly, the synonym for longevity is "length of service." So longevity is also about how much time we have to be in service. Being in service means offering our gifts and our hearts to the world. When we do this, we begin to attract a community of people who are on a similar mission. As we share who we are and recognize our interconnectedness with others, love blossoms. We realize that we are not alone, but we are interconnected. We are one. This generates radiance and joy. Frey, in one of his studies on happiness and longevity, found that happiness extends life by seven-and-a-half to ten years.

From treating and walking hand-in-hand with my patients for many years, I see the true definition of health as moving well beyond being free of disease. It also involves having vital energy, balanced emotions and living a fulfilled, meaningful life. These all generate increased joy, love and radiance, which in turn creates more physical vitality and longevity. I call this approach to health Mindful Medicine where regenerative medicine meets the path of awareness.

With that being said, in my next chapter I will share with you some of my secrets for generating joy in life and true feminine radiance.

Takeaway:

Midlife is a time when both wisdom and experience finally come together. We have cared for our children and put in long hours in our professions. We have finally come to a place in our lives where we can connect to our heart's longing and the interests we long ago sacrificed—a time of passionate new involvement in a life we once dreamed of having. Studies show that happy people live ten years longer. Additional studies show that living one's life's true purpose is an integral part of health and disease prevention.

Picture a guru driving his car to a conference to deliver his messages to millions of people. His car is old and beat up, almost out gas and has only one tire fully inflated. The car breaks down and the guru never makes it to the world summit. Eventually he dies, and all his wisdom and knowledge are never shared. Now, imagine the car is your own body; the 'guru' your essence, wisdom and core spirit. Both need tending or they breakdown. Both can flourish and carry you into very old age where you feel alive and vital, strong and creative, enthusiastic and committed to your mission and the life purpose you have come to fulfill. This is all available to you!

My prescription for your Path of Fulfillment:

- Trust that you have a purpose in life, that you can begin the path to becoming your most expanded and joyous self.

- Be unbridled and courageous in your own self-exploration.

- Allow your purpose to arise from your authentic self.

- Get a time-tested mentor to inspire and guide you, such as Doron Libshtein, Jeffrey Van Dyk, Anil Chandwani or Tim Kelley, who are all dedicated to the evolution of their students.

- Enroll in the "Walk Your Path" webinar on mentorschannel. com.

- Create alliances with others who have similar life missions.

- Through your life purpose, give back to help others.

- Be grateful for the privilege of being the creator of your life.

Chapter 11

The Secret of Feminine Radiance

What prize is earned from having youthful, balanced hormones, a clean-machine body, expanded emotions and a conscious connection to one's "true self"? It is having a special form of radiance permeate and expand you. This radiance exudes an energy that is magnetic. You shine, sizzle, entice and seduce. Regardless of your weight, body type, profession or marital status, people will be drawn you, court you and vie for your attention. I call this integrated state "Feminine Radiance." Not only does it create a magnetic attraction, it also helps create youthful, joyful, robust health. It's a two-way street. A healthy integration of your emotional and conscious self creates vital health. Vital health provides the energy to begin the spiritual journey home to your radiant self.

Having spent thirty years working with women as a hormone specialist, I want to share the insights I have learned about cultivating Feminine Radiance. I started learning these secrets by holding my patients' hands as they passed through traumatic circumstances, adjusting their hormones, and supporting them finding fulfillment in their professions and relationships. I observed them in pain and suffering, and after guiding them in personal growth and healing, I saw them suddenly begin to emanate this distinct type of radiance. I also found many answers from my own experience, as I persistently and passionately embraced my own health and transformation.

By being in the trenches, I have learned there are ten essential steps needed to cultivate Feminine Radiance. Because I want you to understand how to create this for yourself, I have devoted this chapter to that purpose. In thinking about how to best do so—and because so many of my clients ask me about my own life—I decided to use myself as an example. And what do doctors do for their clients? *They write prescriptions.* So each step is offered as a prescription. Fill each one and incorporate all of them into your life, because Feminine Radiance is the inevitable outcome!

As an added step, in the next chapter, there is a super treat: Robin McGraw, one of my dear clients and friends, will share her personal journey to Feminine Radiance. And radiant she has been at every age, inspiring you to be fabulous just like she is.

Let's begin by hanging out together today. It's Saturday morning, and I have just finished my mentoring session with Doron Libshtein. I started mentoring with him two years ago after I took a class on achieving personal dreams. The speaker repeated how important it is to have a mentor to keep you on track with your personal and professional goals. As I thought about the medical training I had undergone for eight years, I realized that becoming a doctor is literally a mentored process. The older, more skilled physicians taught the younger novice medical students and residents their secrets. I thought of all the wonderful physicians who had helped me become who I am today, and immediately decided to work with a mentor again.

Once I made my decision, I wanted to work with the best one I could possibly find. Doron is a mentor to the world's top mentors and our paths had crossed several times over the prior two years. He is frequently in the US, and when I approached him to be my mentor, he sweetly and gently—declined. He simply didn't have the time. He said he was the chairman of too many companies. Looking back, I think he felt I wasn't ready to devote sufficient time to the process due to my demanding schedule.

But I rarely give up, and kept him on my communication radar until he suddenly had a change of heart. He had given up four of his chairman positions and now had time to mentor me. During our very first session, I identified who I truly was and what goals I needed to achieve in the next five years. I wanted to create three new Hall Centers throughout the world. I also wanted to expand my reach to more clients, and realized that I needed to become a speaker. I love to travel and I decided that speaking abroad, and also offering one or two immersion programs a year, would help fulfill that personal goal. Another central purpose I identified was to become a writer. I grew up with a father who was a writer and my little sister, Kathryn, also became a gifted author. It was in my blood too, but I had never identified what I needed to write about or how to begin.

With Doron's mentoring, in my first year I started speaking both in the US and abroad, expanded the Center, created immersion programs and wrote two books. And we discussed and planned every chapter of my books in our sessions. At one of my recent weekly sessions we discussed how to approach the last chapter of this book and our session ended with him cheering me on. "Come on, Prudence," he urged, "you can do this. This is important. Just sit down today and finish it. Finish it so you can help more people. Can you promise this to yourself?"

"Yes! I promise!"

As part of my plan to become a more skilled speaker, I took Brendon Burchard's "The World's Best Speaker Conference," Robert Love's voice class, and Bo Eason's immersion weekend on how to incorporate your personal stories into your talks. I was so inspired by Bo that I joined his Warrior Mastermind group. It is a year-long commitment to accomplish measureable achievable goals. I wanted to become an inspiring speaker for Mindful Medicine and Bo is intense and powerful, instilling a standard of excellence in his students through hard work and unremitting practice.

> ### *The best create the best.*

I can hear Bo now: "Great speakers are not born. They earn it through their commitment, practice and never giving up their dreams."

Who was Bo's acting mentor when he injured himself in the NFL and could no longer play? Al Pacino. He knew that the *best* create the *best*. Indeed, Bo is the most incredible speaker I have experienced, including Tony Robbins.

It is motivating to work with a high-level group, with others who are dedicated, hardworking and high achieving. I also continue working with Doron to expand and refine the Center as well as my additional goals.

My message to you, is you are not alone. You don't have to do it by yourself. You can find mentors who will help you identify and achieve your goals.

Prescription #1

Be committed to your life and be its creative director.
Work with a skilled mentor or become part of a Mastermind group.
Become clear about your objectives and keep moving forward.
Work hard, overcoming any resistance.
Be fabulous on your own unique world stage.

After my sessions with Doron, I always feel happy and inspired. But the current chapter I am working on is complex and I am starting to feel a bit insecure. Will my readers understand what I am trying to convey? I feel self-doubt, worry and even a bit of intimidation. I feel my normal confidence level slip.

I close my eyes and begin addressing this doubting part of myself. Where does this come from? Who is this timid person? After this self-introspection, I realize it comes from concerns about being ridiculed as a bad writer. As soon as I identify this self-doubt, I start laughing. I start to smile, I mean really, how many women are likely to ridicule me for writing this book? Some may not find it interesting, but many will find help and solutions to their problems and feel more confident about how and where to get help. If that happens, the book has succeeded. Besides, I love writing!

> *My path was to be more and more human.*

This brings me to the second step of creating Feminine Radiance. It is so important to be connected to your emotions and feelings. In my family, my father loved British society and told his five children repeatedly that Brits always keep a courageous, stiff upper lip regardless of how they might feel. I wanted to please my father, so I learned to deny what I felt and became a mixture of Pollyanna and a stone Buddha.

As a young adult on a spiritual path I was told, "You are not your emotions." I took that as another confirmation that being unemotional is the way to nirvana. After years of denying my humanness and personal needs, a kind of bitterness arose in me. When I began working with this I was forced to see that my path was not the path of the saint I had longed to become; my path was to be more and more human. With that, I began to allowing myself to feel all the "unnecessary" feelings I had suppressed. I began to cry, be afraid, and feel uncertainty. I experienced jealousy, rage, my own hunger for love and my own insatiability for it. It was a wild ride as I reconnected with the emotions of my humanness, working through years of tears and suppressed humanness within me. My cathartic outpourings allowed the bitterness to leave me and love bloomed once again.

> *Feelings connect us to ourselves. Feelings are messages from our intuition.*

What I have learned from years of stuffing my fears and feelings is that Feminine Radiance is not achieved by pretending we feel something different than we actually do, because it's not more loving; it's not a superior way of being, nor is it good for us. In fact, this kind of pretending chases love away from us because we never share who we truly are. Our fear of vulnerable sharing shuts down the flow of feminine energy. A radiant woman is fully present in life, feeling all aspects of herself and others, as she engages with each moment. She shares herself courageously and lets others know who she actually is. She can use her logic of course, but logic is not the feminine strong suit. It is *knowing* how she feels and sharing herself that allows the energy to flow, creating passion and love. It can feel a bit unsettling in the beginning, feeling emotions flow like a river—sadness, joy, disgust, petulance, anxiety, denial, enthusiasm, affection—and umpteen more feelings, like notes pouring from a flute. Emotions are an important and real step on the path to knowing who you are. Feelings connect us to ourselves, they are messages from our intuition. When we refuse to feel or disown our intuition, we shut down and disconnect from our true selves.

> *Your emotions are your softness, your uniqueness, and your vulnerability, so let yourself be seen.*

Knowing what we value and how we feel about those values allows us to stay true to ourselves. In essence, if we don't know what we value or what we feel, we get confused and can be swayed by what everyone else is saying and feeling. Feeling your emotions doesn't mean you have to act on them or cause harm to others or yourself. It also doesn't mean you have to constantly express them and confuse others around you. But it does mean allowing your feelings to flow freely and not being afraid others will be burdened or upset by them. Truly, your emotions are your softness, your uniqueness, and your vulnerability. Let yourself be seen!

Prescription #2

Experience yourself as an emotional being, including your vulnerability, insatiability, anger, and your tenderness. Don't shut down because it might feel unacceptable. Use your intuition, "your feeling compass." Bring love, encouragement, kindness, compassion, and understanding to yourself. Knowing and loving yourself is a high value.

When negative feelings, self-criticism and despair are persistent, I counsel women to seek professional help. Looking back, I really needed professional help while in my residency. The trauma of caring for sick, dying and destitute patients was worse than I ever could have imagined. I was immersed in the squalor of suffering humanity constantly feeling inadequate and frequently overcome by fears of my own decline and death.

Years later, Ed Gibeau, a truly inspired Jungian analyst, helped me work through much of this. His love and compassionate understanding was absolutely transformational, offering me gentle and humorous insights. Hazel Carter (Indigo Blue) has been another resource. She has brought me a huge appendix of knowledge including EMDR (Eye Movement Desensitization and Reprocessing) and trauma healing. Ger Lyons is another amazing, loving healer. Bringing his Irish intensity to Core Cellular Healing, he offers archangel energy to those in need. During my years of working with him I transformed as I unconditioned core aspects of myself that no longer nourished me. I also have gone to programs in India, taken diverse workshops from Landmark Worldwide, and attended women's groups. I always feel renewed as I discard beliefs and thoughts that no longer serve me. I see each of us as a perfect Michelangelo or Rodin sculpture and by chiseling the unnecessary stone—our conditioning—from the block of granite the beautiful form of the authentic self emerges. And with that, I'd like to give you another prescription.

Prescription #3

Do not ignore your pain; offer yourself the help you need.
When you are no longer growing, you are dying.
Trauma work, therapy, dream analysis and
workshops of all kinds are helpful.
Spiritual teachers, psychologists, analysts, rabbis,
or ministers are all good resources.
Body work, massage, pranic healing, osteopathy,
loving friends are your goldmines.

Speaking of offering yourself help, let's continue the story of my lovely weekend. It is now Saturday night, and I close my eyes to the sound of rain. Rain in Los Angeles! I am cast into my childhood of rainy nights in Oregon. I love to sleep, but I also love the energy of the night. These two desires often conflict and I know I will pay the consequences in the morning if I don't put myself to bed early enough.

During sleep the body detoxifies itself, much like the night cleanup crew. When you sleep six hours or less, the body doesn't get to finish its cycle of cleaning and repair. It can be compared to opening the dishwasher halfway through the cycle and unloading the dirty dishes. Insufficient sleep night after night results in weight gain, memory loss, more depression, wrinkled skin, and a harmed immune system. There is a reason the full eight to nine hours of sleep is appropriately called "beauty sleep"!

I remember times when I had difficulty sleeping, just as many of my patients. I had developed bad insomnia when I was in my medical training and my sleep was all screwed up. I needed to find solutions and ended up teaching myself a form of self-hypnosis. I became so good at it that I learned to fall asleep immediately, anywhere, anytime. I still do this many nights, imagining myself getting lighter and lighter, while being rocked by the sea's waves. I have other techniques as well, which are described next, to rock you into deep sleep.

Prescription #4

Radiant women definitely need to have adequate sleep.
Taking 250-1000 mg of magnesium and
1-2 capsules of Sweet Sleep an hour before bed can be very helpful.
3-10 mg of Melatonin helps if regular sleep is still not achieved
These may be taken separately or all three at once as needed.
Sleep aid meditations are also gloriously helpful.

I love Saturday and Sunday mornings. I frequently sleep until 10:00 or 10:30 and wake up so refreshed. This particular morning

I glance at my phone and see it is only 9:30. Good. I have lots of time. I hop out of bed and I look at myself in the mirror as I pass by and smile. "Good morning, honey," I greet myself in the mirror. I swallow my three grams thyroid supplement, then get in the shower and let the water run over my body. I dry myself enough to slap on some estrogen and testosterone cream to balance my reproductive hormones. I swallow 10,000 IU of the sunshine hormone D3 and two Super Adrenals to keep my adrenal glands strong. Next is my super multi vitamin, Cellular Radiance, and Inflamaleve, a mixture of antioxidants and anti-inflammatories. Hormones and supplements are important, and even I though have given prescriptions for balanced hormones in other chapters, I want to say again—hormonal balance to youthful levels with bioidentical hormones is absolutely essential to creating Feminine Radiance.

Prescription #5

Balance your hormones to youthful levels with bioidentical hormones. Get your tests and lab tests every 6-12 months to remain balanced. Take all of your supplements as they help guard against the major causes of aging and illness.

I make my morning organic, plant-based, sprouted protein shake and start sipping its delicious dense fruit and green mixture. How could I live without my morning smoothie? Food and how we nourish our bodies is so important! At the basis of The Hall Center diet is a morning smoothie, unlimited fresh greens, and vegetables, fruits and berries. They are high in fiber and nutrients. Beans, nuts, seeds, sweet potatoes, quinoa and health oils add even more nutrients and satiety. If you choose to eat meat, then make it an occasional organic animal protein. It is important to eliminate from your diet grains, gluten, sugar, corn, dairy and most animal protein. The Radiant Feminine definitely eats well and it shows!

Prescription #6

Eat The Hall Center Pyramid Diet for greatest energy, strength and beauty.
Don't let your metabolism drop by skipping meals or under-fueling your body.

My morning starts slowly, which is perfect for doing my yoga. I click on an Indian raga I love and slowly center myself. I am wearing my little t-shirt from the night and underwear—perfect yoga attire. I lift my hands up as I breath in, and then lower them as I breath out. My breath moves my arms. I am life's bellows as I breathe in and out with my movements. Now I sweep up like a bird, then down to embrace the ground. I am that movement. Mark Whitwell has been a wonderful teacher for me, a master who sees how each of us is the bloom of life.

On weekdays I practice for about fifteen minutes, but today I am feeling so rested I do thirty minutes. There is no longer a voice in my head telling me I am not doing it right. In these moments I live "out beyond right doing and wrong doing" … in that field of full potential Rumi describes. When I am done, I do my Sadhguru meditation. Sometimes I choose to click on Mentors Channel to do their daily meditation. I have different practices for various days. The reason I keep doing my practices is simple: *they feel so good.* There is no drill sergeant who forces me to step up, be a man and be disciplined. No, it is the lover who seduces me into the sweetness of the experience and the sensitivity of emotions that arise. So here's another piece to our Feminine Radiance puzzle.

Prescription #7

Feminine Radiance is cultivated by practices that connect you to your essential self. They might be chi gong, tai chi, meditation, yoga, mantra chanting, prayer, or other unique forms of connection.

Speaking of the lover, love is a vital ingredient for the recipe of Feminine Radiance. Without the flow of loving energy, feminine nature doesn't thrive. An open, loving heart beacons love. My understanding of this arose over a ten-year period as I travelled to and from India. With each immersion into my spiritual self, I felt a deepening of who I am. As I worked through feelings of being unworthy and unlovable, I began to feel a small light shining within me. As it grew, I identified it as the light of self-love, which grew into a love for all things, including myself.

I began having glimpses of a supreme, almost devotional kind of love that transcends ordinary physical love. In ancient Indian writing from 4000 BC, Radha represents that kind of love with Lord Krishna. Together, they form the blissful union of the masculine and feminine as One. It doesn't matter if you have never been to India, have never read about world religions or

> **Without the flow of loving energy, feminine nature doesn't thrive.**

> *Radiance arises from one who offers and receives love fully.*

even heard of Radha or Krishna. For me, it was simply a feeling of knowing that I was the Beloved, that my path was one of supreme, devotional love. It was the experience of no separation between love and myself—only light and love everywhere. My breath became One with everything, my soul became all souls. One is love. One is peace. One is joy. One is everywhere.

I now see how we enter into a state of grace through our practices and by our desire to unite with Source by knowing that we are one with Source. Whether it is the experience of devotional, pure love as I experience it, or love as you experience it, love is an essential aspect of the Radiant Feminine. Radiance arises from one who offers and receives love fully. In fact, it arises from *being* love.

Prescription #8

Union as the Beloved
Experience unending union with yourself, your Source,
your beloved, moment-by-moment. Never separate.

Community is very important to me, as it is for most women. I like a lively, multitalented group made up of teacher-gurus, artists, philosophers, "characters" and family. This Saturday, my friend Tony Cronin is texting me and wants to swing by for tea. I get ready and greet him at the front door. After we sit down he is full of ideas for his next play. He started a Westside LA Shakespeare troupe called "Colonials." Should he put on *Merchant of Venice or*

Twelfth Night for his next play? A good discussion ensues. I love his long dialogues about Shakespeare's finer points, as he quotes Hamlet, or the tortured Romeo. My son Conrad drops by for gluten-free waffles with his sweet girlfriend, Alex. They join in the conversation. Conrad is Romeo with his Juliet and understands what Tony is saying. Susanna, one of my wonderful friends and practitioners at the Center, drops by with news of the clinic. It will be a busy day tomorrow.

I love being part of this multi-dimensional community. The Radiant Feminine has her entourage of friends, colleagues, and family. She inspires others and is inspired. She gives and receives in a seamless flow. She leads and is led.

Prescription #9

Community: take time for friends, kids, family.
Do communal activities, talking, cooking, working and playing together.
Help when there is need—and receive help.

It is Sunday and I visited a friend in the hospital. Only thirty-two years old, he has received a diagnosis of cancer and has gone through hellish surgery. Today he is sitting up in bed, off all pain medication, with tears welling in his eyes.

"Prudence, this is the best thing that has ever happened to me. I am just so grateful. I knew I was off base with my work, and for the last six months I have been praying for something to release me back to my real life's purpose. And the whole time I have been here, so sick for the last eight days, I didn't think once—not even once—about money, my current work, the deals I am doing or anything else. The only thing that is important to me is love—my mother, friends, those who came to visit—only about love. So my prayers came true. This cancer, which of course I'm going to survive, has put me back on course and now I can begin the second part of my life—the real part that I've waited this long to start. I am going to be in service and help others. I am so grateful I have been given this chance to see myself and make the changes I needed to make. Some people die without having the chance to do what they came to do."

> *Gratitude is generated by realizing that nothing happens to me; it happens for me.*

We both have tears in our eyes, and I am so grateful to receive this teaching from one who has been severely tried.

My weekend has meandered slowly to Sunday night, and I fall asleep with my eye pillow over my eyes. The rain has stopped and before I drift off, I ask myself what is holding all these prescriptions together? As I drift into sleep, I feel one of the essential elements: gratitude. Gratitude moves us from being victims in our lives, to receiving life's gifts. Gratitude is generated by realizing that nothing happens *to* me; it happens *for* me—even bad divorces, losing our jobs, or having money embezzled, which happened to me. Everything is ultimately *for us, not against us.*

Prescription #10

Gratitude
Gratitude is a state of mind.
Do a two-minute practice of feeling gratitude each morning and
evening.
Use gratitude whenever depressed, sad, or in doubt.

Every stream I have followed in my life has been a gift. Each event has helped me create radiance in my life—all the suffering, hard work, marriages, children, friends, travels, community, spiritual practices, and love. Feminine Radiance is cultivated by the grace of manifestation and transformation. We create Life; we are Life. We cannot escape it because it is simply and fully who we are. We can live as unbridled beings of light and love, freely and joyfully, or we can work hard to block it. It is an urgent choice, and it has an expiration date.

Some women pass so deeply into despair they cannot return. You must not hold back, even if in the moment you are alone and feel you have nothing to offer. You do, and you don't have to figure it out all by yourself. Just fill the prescriptions I have given you and get help whenever resistance comes up. Surely we can't live without guidance or the expertise of others. Balancing your hormones can be quick and easy. Healing past trauma is the beginning of a fascinating journey, and as you get to know your life purpose more clearly, your community will begin to form around you. Others will begin to recognize you, as they did me, and will join to help you. Radiance attracts radiance, and suddenly you will look up and realize you are in love with your life, and in joy with your own exploration.

> *Feminine Radiance is cultivated by the grace of manifestation and transformation.*

Chapter 12

Revelations from Radiant Robin McGraw

For this last chapter I wanted to select a woman whose life story would inspire and guide on their path to Feminine Radiance. Robin McGraw, a dear friend and client, is that woman. Robin emanates the full beauty and power of Feminine Radiance, and her razor sharp understanding of herself and life has made her a role model for millions of women worldwide. She is one of the most positive and authentic people I know, along with being wise, funny, and a fabulous storyteller. Filled with a desire to help alleviate all human suffering, she also has a special place in her compassionate heart for women who suffer.

Not only has Robin been a daily presence on the Dr. Phil show since its inception in 2002, she has appeared on the Oprah Winfrey Show, The Doctors, and has cohosted many other television productions. Robin is a highly sought after public speaker, a two-time New York Times best-selling author. She is a board member of The Dr. Phil Foundation for mental health and the founder of When Georgia Smiled, Robin McGraw Revelation. Robin has devoted her life to a wide variety of philanthropic organizations. As a wife, mother, and grandmother, she radiates feminine love and wisdom.

In the interview that follows, Robin generously shares her life's challenges and the revelations that have transformed her. Dear readers, it is my joy to introduce you to Robin McGraw—courageous, unbridled, and uniquely herself.

Prudence: What makes you who you are—this radiant, positive, and loving woman? What influenced you to become this person? There's not another Robin in the whole world like you!

Robin: That's true, because there is not another one of any of us anywhere. We are all our own person. One thing that has helped create the woman I am today is that I've always believed in being educated, and aware of myself in every way possible. Whenever anything would affect me physically or interest me mentally, or if something affected my family or close friends, I would do everything I could to educate myself in order to get answers to all of my questions. I love reading, studying, and stimulating my brain with every bit of information I can find.

That is the path I took when I started menopause. I would go to the library and read everything I could find on hormones. I also went to bookstores and studied each book before deciding which one to buy. I visited pharmacies and spoke with the pharmacists. I made appointments with brilliant doctors like you, Prudence, and asked all of my questions. It's of utmost importance to educate yourself and to know your body so you can help yourself. Figure out the questions you want to know about your body, then go ask the experts for answers. No one knows your body like you do.

You know how it feels when you eat something that isn't good for you? I now know I can't handle dairy or seafood, but I had to pay attention and care, or else I wouldn't have known that. So you have to learn about your body. For example, when I began to experience menopause, I didn't recognize what was happening.

Prudence: You were around 40?

Robin: I had started feeling changes within myself at 40, but the symptoms got really intense when my son, Jay, was about to leave for college when I was 42. I would find myself taking some time to reflect over the years of raising him and preparing him for this new phase of his life. I was very proud of Phillip and myself about how we raised and prepared him for this major milestone in his life. However, there would be times when I would be fatigued, or have midafternoon headaches, and insomnia. At first I told myself it was normal to feel this way, because I was in a big personal transition with Jay going away to college. But when my symptoms continued and even worsened, I realized something else was happening.

The first doctor I saw said, "You are in menopause, and life as you know it is over."

I was shocked that she would say such a thing to me and replied, "Why? Am I dying?"

She wanted to put me on synthetic hormones and she made menopause sound so horrible. She told me to "fill these prescriptions and come back in six months."

I thought, *No!* Then I went home that day and started my campaign to learn everything I could about menopause.

Prudence: Did you learn about bioidentical hormones?

Robin: Yes, but I first learned about every prescription she gave me. What was crazy was that the last one was for Prozac. I didn't want to take any of it! So I got busy and learned what I actually needed was bioindenticals—not the synthetic hormones.

Prudence: And they've given you vitality and renewed good health?

Robin: I feel great! Absolutely vital, healthy, and full of life; and if I have any problems, I call you, Prudence. But really, it was nonsense what the other doctor told me about my life being over. In fact, life is getting better and better all the time. I really helped myself recover quickly through education and staying on top of all the issues.

Prudence: These are such helpful observations about your menopausal journey. I want all women to approach their hormonal transitions with intelligence and curiosity like you've done. I love that you were an advocate for yourself with such a huge transition as menopause. It really paid off.

Robin: It certainly did, and I encourage all women to use this time to get to know themselves better, reclaim their health, and redefine what makes them happy. The second half of life has the possibility of offering us tremendous satisfaction and joy.

Prudence: Can you share other influences on your life and ways of approaching challenges?

Robin: I have been asked this question a lot, and I've even had people challenge who I am, saying things like, "No one is as happy as you are all the time. Every time I see you, you're always smiling. There is just no way someone is this happily married, or this happy with her life." It's as though they're telling me, "You're hiding something, or else you're being fake." But that's not true. Even if I am not *always* feeling happy, or if my marriage is going through challenging times of growth, I *make a choice* to be happy and grateful for the life I have. The way I live my life is a response to my choices. In fact, everything we do in life is a choice. To share what has influenced my life in more depth, I need to go back to my childhood and youth.

I'll start with Phillip asking me to marry him. I told him, "If we're going to do this, we're going to do it and have fun. I agree to be married, but we're not just going to be 'married'—we're going to make the choice to be *happily* married."

People ask, "What gave you that attitude? What made you feel you could say that?"

Well, I've had to think about that. If he and I were still living in Texas as an unknown couple—not like now when countless people on the streets recognize us—I would still be the same person I am right now sitting in front of you. I would still have this personality, this type of outlook on life. It has *nothing* to do with the fact we live in California now, or that my husband has the number one talk show on daytime TV. It has nothing to do with our station in life. It truly has to do with how I choose to respond to what happens to me in life—the choices I make about how I want to live, which began in my childhood.

I can remember my youngest years and people who influenced me, such as my twin brother. We are the youngest of five children. There were three older sisters—three, five and seven years old—before my brother and I arrived. I remember asking my parents if they knew they were having twins and they told me, "No, we didn't." We're talking sixty-two years ago, when there were no ultrasounds. But they did do an X-ray because my mother was feeling unusual pain on one side of her stomach. However, they didn't know they were having twins until the last minute.

We were born two months premature, and the only thing they saw on the X-ray was three feet! I was born first, another daughter after having three girls already at home. My brother was born five minutes later and I'd say that shaped who I am. When you're one of a multiple birth, there is something very unique about that. I believe I was born first so I could tell my brother, "Come on out now," as well as what to do and how to do it. Truly, I've been taking care of him my whole life. Because of my twin brother, I believed that I would love giving birth to all boys. Interestingly enough, that came true: Phil and I have two sons. So who I was going to become started at birth. Another influence on my life was my middle sister, with whom I am particularly close. I love all my sisters, but she really helped shape the person I am today.

The most important influence happened one pivotal night when I was twelve years old. I can honestly tell you the very night I lay in bed and decided the kind of woman I would become, the wife I would become, and the mother I would be. However, I want to share a little more of my background first.

Growing up we were very poor. My father was an alcoholic, and when he drank he gambled. We had nothing and certainly nothing to gamble with. But he was an amazing golfer, so he would make bets on the golf course. He was also a car salesman with the gift of charm. But in spite of doing a pretty good job, we were poor. He would leave the house every Sunday morning and we'd all hold our breath to see if he would show up that night. The darker it got, the more we'd be listening for his car. Many Sundays we went to bed without him coming home. No one talked about it, because truly we all adored him and he adored my mother. He really thought he was doing us a favor by not drinking in front of us, but there was a cost. If he made the choice on a Sunday to get drunk and play cards at some municipal golf course and not show up for dinner, we knew he wasn't coming home that night.

I lived a life of uncertainty, which also shaped me growing up. I never knew when my father would come home, or if we would have enough money to pay bills or buy food. Honestly, we never knew how long one of his benders would last. We knew when one was over because he'd come home, close the bedroom door, shower, and sleep it off. My father was very meticulous about his appearance and never wanted us to see him intoxicated. I couldn't bring friends home because it might be awkward if they'd ask, "Where's your dad? Why is it so quiet in here? Why is everyone tiptoeing around?" That was tough on all of us.

The one certain and positive part of my life, the one person I knew I could count on was my mother, Georgia. She was unwavering in her dedication to make our lives the easiest and safest she could. And she always had a beautiful smile on her face. She knew the five of us children were uncertain about our day-to-day life when my dad was drinking, but I could look to her for support. She would smile—and I'm talking about a smile that was not only on her lips but one that came from her eyes. I could feel it from her heart. It was powerful. It was magical. My mother was the one person who got me through my childhood—her strength, her support, and her smile. Her smile would make me feel as if life were great. It said that everything was going to be okay, everything was going to be just fine. Her smile was the only thing that would help me go to sleep at night.

All of this affected and shaped me, but there is one particular incident that really impacted me when I was twelve. I was alone with my mother that night. We had a very small tract home throughout which you could hear everything. I was in my room sleeping, when about three in the morning I heard this banging. I thought it was a tornado!

As I became fully awake, I realized someone was banging on the front door and I thought, *This can't be Dad. He's never done anything like this.* I scrambled out of bed and ran through the tiny living room, only to see my five-foot-four-inch-tall mother standing in the open doorway with a cotton robe pulled around her. Three men stood on the other side, and they were really drunk.

Mom said, "What are you doing here?"

"We've come for what is ours, for what belongs to us," one of them replied.

She asked, "What are you talking about? Where is Jim?" (That's my father.)

"He's not with us," another said.

I knew that we were both thinking, *Why did my dad let these people come to our house? He had to have told them where we lived.*

My mother looked up and asked them, "What are you here for? What are you talking about?"

"We came to collect all your furniture that we won in a poker game."

I was just in shock! I was thinking, *My dad did this? He gave all our furniture away in a poker game and sent these men to collect it?* I stood there shaking in quiet disbelief that this was happening.

Then I looked at my mother who stood up straighter; she seemed to grow to be 10 feet tall and 500 pounds. I'll never forget it. She looked at those men with her back very straight, staring them right in the eye—three big men and my little mother facing them. They could have knocked down our cardboard door! I thought they were coming right in and would take me too, or whatever they wanted.

But my mother stood there and said, "You're not coming into my home, and you're not taking anything that belongs to me. You need to go home and have your wives call me in the morning, and *we'll* discuss what belongs to you." Then she shut the door and put the chain in the lock. Even though they could have knocked the door down with a flick of a finger, they walked away.

My mother turned around and looked at me. I don't know how she knew I was standing there the entire time, but she then said,

"Everything's going to be okay. Now you go to sleep, sweetheart." She then turned around and walked into her bedroom and shut the door. She left me by myself, but she had smiled at me and comforted me.

I don't know how long I stood there, but I remember going back to my bedroom and not getting a wink of sleep that night. As I lay there in my bed, that night was a pivotal time in my life. So much went through my mind: my father could do that; those men could do that. But one thing I will never forget is how strong my mom's voice was when her back stiffened and she authoritatively told those men, "You go home and tell your wives to call me in the morning." She *knew* those women wouldn't let them take our furniture because they also were married to alcoholics and knew exactly what she was going through—they were all going through it too.

That was the first lesson that came to me: *Women stick together.* They were married to alcoholics just like she was, and they would support each other. That night I made some monumental decisions that would define the rest of my life. I decided right then and there, "I will never marry a man who drinks alcohol, and when I am blessed with children, I will not raise them in a home with an alcoholic father. It will not happen!"

I have to say that the first date I had with Phillip, I asked him, "Do you drink alcohol?"

"Do you know what?" he replied, "I don't, because I think I am allergic to it."

I thought, *I think I love this man already.* But of course that's not what made me fall in love with him, but it sure was the first step, because I stuck by what I decided that night when I was a child. That night taught me so much and defined who I am. My mother taught me about the strength and resolve of a woman. When I stood behind her and saw her make a decision to protect the little we had, to defend her home and family against those three men, I knew right then I would be just like her. When I had a family and when I had a home, I would do whatever it took to protect all of us. I have lived by that decision every day. I would *never* allow those I love to suffer and be scared. I told myself that I would have a smile on my face every day because I knew what a smile brought to my life—peace and comfort. I knew that I would live my life with a smile coming from my heart, from my eyes and voice, and every bit of my soul would go into it—for my children, my husband, or anyone who needed it, including people I didn't even know. When people say, "There's no way you can be that happy all the time," maybe I'm not happy in that moment, but it is a choice for me to do whatever I can to help myself and anyone who might need my encouragement.

I never knew we would leave Texas and come to California, then become well known because of the Dr. Phil Show. But I thank God for where we are today, because I have been able to create When Georgia Smiled, The Robin McGraw Revelation Foundation, and help women and children who suffer from domestic violence.

Many people ask, "Have you suffered from domestic violence?"

I respond, "No."

"Has your mother?"

I tell them no. I wasn't abused physically, but because of the disease my father had which he could not overcome, there were countless times when I needed comfort and strength. I hope to reach out and give both to whomever is in need—men, women, and children. That kind of support is how I got through my childhood. My father didn't make choices in his life, the illness made his choices. He did whatever he could to keep us from suffering. Even though he didn't drink around us, or come home drunk, throughout our childhood all of us kids suffered.

Prudence: Can you tell us more about your Foundation?

Robin: My reason for focusing on domestic violence is because I've sat through every show Phillip has taped, and the ones that moved me the most were about people who sought help for domestic violence. You might think I would have been more touched by the shows about alcoholism, but I wasn't; I was touched by the women, along with their children, who needed to get out of their physically violent relationships.

It's not just women who are violated—it's men too. Those brave men and women who had suffered from domestic violence would come back to help those who were still suffering. They had the courage and the strength to want to reach out and help because they were able to extricate themselves. I thought, *Amazing! You've suffered so much yourself, yet here you are helping others who are suffering.* They offered that same sense of peace, love, support, and comfort my mother gave me when she smiled, so I named the foundation When Georgia Smiled, wanting to give them that same peace I received.

I am very proud of the Foundation. I am very proud of the products we sell with 100 percent of the net proceeds going back to the Foundation. We've given numerous grants to shelters all over the country. We launched it along with the Aspire Initiative, which is a program on our site that helps people in abusive relationships educate themselves. Individuals can access the Aspire Initiative with family or on their own, and it's being used across the country in afterschool programs and at many civic centers. Sometimes people don't even know they're in an abusive relationship, simply because they've been in it their entire lives. We teach the warning signs, what to do, and how to get help.

We also help people to know if they are an abuser. They might not even know they are an abuser because they have been abused their entire lives—abuse is all they know. An abuser hits someone once and says, "I didn't mean to do that. Come back." In my opinion, communication through violence is abusive, and perpetrators need help.

We help people identify whether or not they are dating or are married to an abuser. Aspire Initiative is filled with tests and programs. It's a beautiful site where you can educate yourself and education is so key for the eradication of domestic violence.

We also have created the ASPIRE app, and I am so proud of this! It has been downloaded more than 350,000 times around the world. We also have over fifteen different news sites such as

USA today, CNN, and LA Opinion. When an abuser takes your phone, he/she sees what looks like a normal news site. But when you tap a stripe across the top of the app, it takes you into the app, which is where you can find help. It contacts three or four pre-designated friends, family members, or coworkers who are your emergency contacts. Let's say you're being abused—when you hit the stripe at the top of the app, your contacts are notified with your prerecorded message or a text and know to come and rescue you.

There is also a GPS tracking device on the app, so if the abuser takes you away from the house your contacts will know where to find you. Your message will even go to 911 if you desire. Finally, there is a recording device in the app that records without a red light blinking, allowing you to record what is happening. Abusers frequently tell the police that you started the fight and that *you* are the abuser, not the victim. I am proud to say that when we launched this app, it was recognized on Capital Hill as one of the two best apps in the country for educating people on domestic violence.

Robin: Another influence or revelation that formed me when I was a young woman took place right when Phillip and I moved into a really old house. We planned to renovate and update it a bit, and I still recall the musty smell it had. My fifty-eight-year-old mother was with us that night, helping unload boxes. Near the middle of the night she said, "Sweetheart, I'm going home, and I'll come back tomorrow to help you unpack more."

I replied, "Before you come over, would you just make me a pumpkin pie?" She was a phenomenal cook and I loved her pumpkin pies.

"I would love that," she said.

The next day, she called to tell me she had just taken the pie out of the oven. I was happy thinking about how good it would smell in a house that was kind of musty. We hung up, and then she called back shortly after and asked if Phil was home.

"No, he went to the grocery store," I responded. "He's picking up some bread and milk for breakfast. Why? What do you need?"

"Oh, I just wanted to ask him something. I'm feeling kind of funny."

"What do you mean by funny?" I asked.

The phone went dead.

"Mother? Mother!"

No answer. I thought because we were in an old house and it had been raining, the connection was bad. I hung up just as Phillip came through the back door. He stepped into the kitchen and the phone rang again.

"Oh that's my mother," I said. "She called for you, but we got disconnected."

When he picked up the phone, I heard screaming in the background. I heard him ask her, "Have you called an ambulance?" then quickly assert, "We're coming right over."

"What was that about?" I asked.

"Well, your mother fell over on the bed. That's why the phone got disconnected."

Now I know how to read Phillip, so I was alarmed. We raced over and ran back to the bedroom. She was there on the bed and already turning blue. Phillip started doing CPR and I ran out to the front yard because I heard the ambulance sirens.

Mom was soon on a stretcher, then loaded into the ambulance. Phillip asked if I wanted to ride with my mother. I got in, but her monitor went off with a shriek and I tore out of the ambulance to ride with Phil. I'll never forget how slow the ambulance was going—and they weren't running the siren. I kept asking myself, *Why aren't they going faster? Why don't they have the siren on?*

When we got to the hospital, Phillip came back to tell me, "She's gone. She didn't make it."

I'll never forget looking at him saying, "It can't be. It just can't be. Why, she's never even been to the doctor!"

That's when I had my revelation. She never went to a doctor a day in her life, and that's why she wasn't with us. She never put *herself* first. She put us first. She never took care of herself. If we needed to go to the doctor, she took us. It was always about someone else, but never about herself. That was my revelation! I thought, *She just taught me a valuable lesson on the day of her death.* I told myself, *I will perpetuate her legacy in every way, but not with this one thing. I will not perpetuate her legacy of self-neglect.*

It was that day I knew I wanted to be around for my children to grow up. I wanted to be with my husband for the rest of my long life. And because of my mother's sudden death, I saw I needed to take care of myself first. I needed to put myself at the top of my list. To this day I always say, "If you don't put yourself first, you're teaching everyone to put you second," and that is a shame!

Prudence: That's right! So many women don't even put themselves second. They put themselves last.

Robin: That is not okay. It doesn't pay to be a martyr. You have to say, "I come first." Yes, the Lord comes first—that's a given. But if you don't put yourself next, you won't be there to help the ones you love. Who's going to take care of them if you're gone?

My dear mother should have known that it's not selfish to take care of yourself, because then you're putting the love of your family at the top of the list. You will be there for those you love. You will see them grow up. If you love yourself enough, you will put yourself first.

When my grandson, Jordan, was three years old, I had another revelation. Whenever my son, Jay, his wife, Erica, and their two children would come over, I always stood on the front porch as they drove up. It was my little ritual, waiting for them to get out of the car.

One day my grandson jumped out of the car and said, "Where's your car, Grandma? Where's your car?"

"It's in the garage. Do you want to see it?"

"I want to see it!" he exclaimed.

But I just stopped right there, and as I looked at that darling little face I thought, *I'm so glad I took the time to put myself at the top of the list so I can be here, listening to his voice saying to me, "Grandma, where's your car?"*

My mother died one year to the day before our youngest son was born. She never got to hear him say, "Grandma, I'm gonna grow up one day and learn to play the guitar; I'll learn to sing; I'm going to have a band; and I may even win a Grammy one day."

He never got to hear her say, "I know that you will, baby. I know you will."

Look at what both of them missed. If she had gone to the doctor, even once, who knows where life would have taken her. My message is this: It's never too late to start taking care of yourself because if you don't, you will miss out on so many precious moments.

The day I had that revelation changed my life. I love my family, and I'm going to take care of myself.

Prudence: When you talk about how you've put yourself first, I see it includes physically *and* emotionally.

Robin: When I make a decision, it's all or nothing. I've been that way my whole life. When I make a decision, in my heart I know it's what I need. As I shared earlier, when we got married, I said we're going to have fun. We're not going to be *just* married; we're going to be *happily* married. People don't believe it when Phillip and I say we never fight. I have never in forty-four years, including forty years of marriage, raised my voice at him. I've never screamed or shouted. I just don't. It's not necessary. I'm not going to be in a marriage where I have to scream at my partner. He doesn't want to live like that either. We have rules, and we told each other our needs and our wants before we got married.

Prudence: Throughout your enduring relationship with Phillip you have not sacrificed your physical beauty. So many women sacrifice their self-care when they become a mother, or a grandmother, but you haven't.

Robin: I have said this many times before: I believe that I was put on this earth to be a grandmother. The ultimate reward now is being a grandmother. I can't say enough how much I love it. I love being a grandmother! I love it, I love it, I love it!

Prudence: You once told me people are always telling you to dress your age.

Robin: Yes they do! Dress my age? My mental age, or a number? Let me tell you, my numerical age has never been an issue for me. When I see something I love, I'm going to wear it. We're all smart enough to know what we look and feel good in, and that's what I'm going to wear.

Just because I'm sixty-two doesn't mean I'm going to wear a certain type of clothing or style or my hair a certain way. No! I'm going to wear my clothes and my hairstyle in a way that makes me feel good. You could be the ripest, juiciest peach in the whole world, but there's always going to be someone who doesn't like peaches.

There's something I do with the women on my staff that they think is funny. I reach up and pretend to adjust my crown, so they'll remember they're wearing one too. Every woman deserves to wear a crown.

Prudence: What would you like to leave with our readers to help each of them be fabulous and radiant?

Robin: I encourage all women to do what it takes to live their happiest and healthiest life. Learn who you are from the inside out. Learn what your body needs and what you need emotionally so you can live with radiance and vitality. It takes some time alone with yourself to discover who you are and what you need, whether it is through prayer, by writing in your journal, reading, taking a walk. I want you to know you are precious and worth it, and don't let anyone ever tell you that you aren't. Wake up every day to live a life of peace and joy and find contentment with the unique and fabulous person you are. You deserve it!

Prudence: Thank you for sharing your wisdom with our readers, dear Robin. Your courage shines through every aspect of your life. Your love and devotion is obvious, and so is your joy of being in service to your community and the world. I do believe every aspect of your life contributes to your shining radiance. You have done it, my dear, and now you are helping others become centered, powerful, and radiant too. My heart is filled with gratitude.

FINAL Words

Just as each river seeks its ocean source, you too are on a journey back to the source of who you are. The journey back to yourself involves recognizing when you get off course, and then getting back on again. If my clients in this book hadn't recognized what was happening to them and then decided to take action, they would still be suffering and causing suffering to those around them. It wasn't always easy for them to stop and assess what was happening, but this is the first step. It took courage to commit to themselves, balance their hormones, change their lifestyle and dive into the tender interior of emotional balance. I sometimes wish life happened in the bleachers where we could simply be a spectator. But it doesn't. It happens on the field where there are rough calls and some very hard knocks. When we commit to our life-game with authenticity and sincerity, a wonderful thing happens. The pain and suffering we've experienced creates compassion and greater love for ourselves and others. These are necessary ingredients for creating a meaningful life of purpose and fulfillment.

Many women who have suffered are now full of life again. Perhaps you saw yourself in one of their stories. You are not alone. Join with me, Robin McGraw, Suzanne Somers, Karina Stewart, Doron Libshtein, and all the women and men in this book who have shared their stories. Join us and we'll add to your strength, just as you'll add to ours. With each person who goes before us, the path home becomes more illuminated and clear. As we journey together rather than saying with despair, "I simply don't recognize who I am anymore," you will joyfully say, "I love this passionate, vital person I am becoming!" Then all the heavens will smile, for it will be clear who you are. You are the radiance of your unique, loving, wise, and beautiful self exactly as you were meant to be.

With love to each of you,

Prudence

Now that you have walked with other women on their way back to health,

It's time for you!

Which of your hormones are imbalanced and what can be done to correct them?

What needs to be changed in your life so you can live your fuller vision?

Our accurate analyses and the education you receive are precisely tailored to you.

Be your radiant, vital self by taking this first step to learn about our online programs. Please visit:

www.radiantagain.com